Praise from the Expe

"This book fills a niche—it is difficult to find specific guidance on programming validation. Often, what can be found is very complicated and not directly applicable to SAS programming in the pharmaceutical industry. Carol and Brian have consolidated a lot of information about clinical trial data report validation and presented it in a way that makes it accessible and usable by programmers at all levels.

"This book provides a straightforward, concrete plan for meeting the complex validation requirements that clinical trial data reporting must adhere to. By including actual sample validation checklists in the book's appendix, the authors have allowed readers to implement the suggestions in the book with just a little effort."

Kim Truett
KCT Data, Inc.

"Having taught a pharmaceutical-focused SAS programming class since 1998 using two other SAS Press publications, I am thrilled to say that this book will be such a benefit to my class as well as to others in the industry. The information it contains is 100% applicable to the tasks associated with clinical trial reporting. I recommend this book to SAS programmers just entering the pharmaceutical industry, as well as to those that have years of experience in the industry. There are some wonderful nuggets in this book!"

Daphne Ewing
Sr. Director, Programming
Auxilium Pharmaceuticals, Inc.

"For programmers who are relatively new to the industry or for those who have long been part of it, Carol and Brian's book provides a good overview, practical hands-on tips, and many examples of how to perform a thorough validation. The authors' written style allows the reader to almost see and hear Carol and Brian sitting nearby in conversation.

"The SAS programming examples in the book are very clear and easy to follow. This is a good reference book for all statistical and clinical SAS programmers."

Susan Fehrer
President
BioClin, Inc.

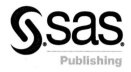

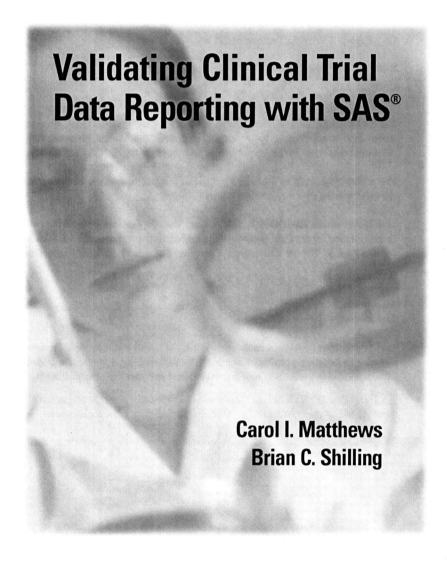

Validating Clinical Trial Data Reporting with SAS®

Carol I. Matthews
Brian C. Shilling

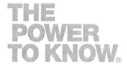

The correct bibliographic citation for this manual is as follows: Matthews, Carol I., and Brian C. Shilling. 2008. *Validating Clinical Trial Data Reporting with SAS*®. Cary, NC: SAS Institute Inc.

Validating Clinical Trial Data Reporting with SAS®

Copyright © 2008, SAS Institute Inc., Cary, NC, USA

ISBN 978-1-59994-128-8

Contents

Preface

Validation of a SAS programmer's work is of the utmost importance in any industry. It is of even greater importance in the pharmaceutical industry. Because the pharmaceutical industry is governed by federal laws, SAS programmers are bound by a very strict set of rules and regulations. These rules and regulations are defined and enforced to ensure that the information presented to the Food and Drug Administration (FDA) on a single clinical trial or on a set of trials is accurate. Reporting accuracy is crucial because these data represent people, the patients or subjects of the trials. The well-being, quality of life and, above all, safety of these people are represented and reported by these data.

There are many ways that SAS can be used throughout the clinical trial process—ad-hoc reports tracking the status of clinical data, data edit checks, analysis data sets, and summary tables. Depending on the task, the validation requirements can be more or less stringent. While SAS can be used for any number of tasks, the vast majority of these tasks involve the final analysis and reporting of the clinical trial data. While each of these tasks is unique, the SAS tools that are used to produce each of them are very similar—the DATA step and a variety of procedures, such as PROC SORT, PROC PRINT, and PROC FREQ, are used to manipulate data and produce an end result. So, this book first discusses the general concepts that apply to almost any programming task and then addresses items that are specific to either the task or the type of data with which you work. While the validation techniques discussed in this book can be applied to almost any type of programming, the main focus is on validating programs that import and export data from different file types; programs that create analysis data sets; and programs that create summary tables, data listings, and figures.

Validation is integral to many aspects of the programming process for clinical trials. Defining validation and discussing how to do it are often difficult. Validation can refer to syntax (is the code itself doing what it was intended to do?), the underlying data being manipulated (does the data contain what we expect and does the data behave the way we expect?), or the final result produced by the code (does the result make sense?). While in most cases it is relatively easy to check the syntax (the SAS log is very useful for this purpose), checking the data and the final output are often much more difficult. These latter aspects of validation also require experience to understand what to check and how.

There are several ways to discuss what a programmer needs to know to effectively validate SAS programs in the pharmaceutical industry. There are general, guiding principles about how to approach the issue, such as whether to validate through independent programs or through peer reviews. Beyond that, there are several general coding techniques you can use to validate specific types of code. For example, any time you program a frequency distribution, you can create a cell index, as discussed in Chapter 4.

Critical to effective validation is the programmer's understanding of the data with which they will be working. If you don't understand how the data is arranged, the values that are reasonable for each variable, and the way the data should behave, you will not ensure that the specifications are complete or even appropriate. Often programmers have difficulty finding a company willing to hire them without pharmaceutical experience. Companies know that understanding the data makes a huge difference in a programmer's effectiveness. Good programmers can program output to match specifications; exceptional programmers evaluate the specifications as they program and provide valuable input to the process as a whole.

Another key piece involved in validation is purely technical. As most experienced programmers know, there are usually at least two ways in SAS to obtain a given result. A good programmer should know multiple methods to arrive at the same result to ensure that the result is truly correct.

Because validation is so integral to programming, it can be difficult to find a beginning and an end to a conversation on this topic. This book starts with an outline of the general industry standards and expectations, which are in large part the driving forces behind validation. Subsequent chapters address general validation concepts, followed by chapters detailing items to look for in the major data topics as well as different methods to calculate similar items that are frequently programmed. This book also assumes that the reader has at least a general understanding of the pharmaceutical industry and focuses on how to validate output rather than how to create that output in the first place. If you are completely new to this industry and need a better understanding of how SAS is applied in general, we recommend Jack Shostak's book *SAS Programming in the Pharmaceutical Industry*.

As you read this book, you will notice that it contains many acronyms, not all of which are standard throughout the industry. Refer to Appendix C, Glossary, if you are not sure what an acronym or industry term means.

Acknowledgments

After several years of writing, rewriting, editing, and review, our manuscript regarding the validation of clinical trial data reporting is finally a reality. We could not have completed the text within these covers without the direction, assistance, dedication, and perseverance of numerous individuals. For all of your hard work and guidance during this process, we would like to thank the reviewers who skillfully helped us to mold our text into its final form: Annette Bove, Sue Carroll, Brent Cohen, David Handelsman, Neil Howard, Maria Keyser, Angela Lightfoot, Gene Lightfoot, Hunter McGhee, Andy Ravenna, Jack Shostak, and David Wiehle.

We would like to extend our warmest thanks to Ms. Katy White, our colleague at United BioSource Corporation. Katy was instrumental in the review and editing of our text and managed to help us give it a united voice. Thank you Katy—your input was invaluable!

We would also like to thank the SAS editing and production team that worked so closely with us and kept us motivated during the challenging times. Thank you to Mary Beth Steinbach, our managing editor; Kathy Restivo and Joel Byrd, our copyeditors; Candy Farrell and Monica McClain, our technical publishing specialists; Patrice Cherry and Jennifer Dilley, our designers; and Shelly Goodin and Liz Villani, our marketing specialists. At the top of our SAS "thank you" list is Judy Whatley, our acquisitions editor. We owe Judy so much more than a thank you! We greatly appreciate all of the time, patience, and perseverance that you exercised during the years of work and updates this text has gone through. You have been our touchstone during the entire process and we thank you dearly.

We would be remiss if we didn't mention all of our coworkers and colleagues that we used as "lab rats" while writing the book. Our deepest gratitude to all of our colleagues and friends at United BioSource Corporation, BioCor, Covance, and all of the other great companies for whom we have had the pleasure of working.

In closing, we would like to thank our families for letting us use their nights and weekends to work on this project, and for having to listen to us talk about it, and talk about it … and talk about it some more for the past few years. Thanks to Carol's family (Cullen, Allie, and Riley) for all of the missed or delayed family outings and game nights; thanks to Brian's parents (Nancy and Charlie) for being a tireless sounding board for the past 5 years. Without all of your support, we never could have done it —just saying thank you doesn't seem adequate!

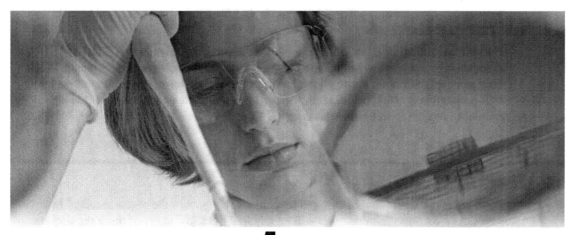

C h a p t e r 1

Pharmaceutical Industry Overview

1.1 Introduction

The pharmaceutical industry, including clinical research organizations (CROs) and biotechnology companies, has adopted many industry standards and requirements. While these standards affect the entire clinical trial process, many have a direct impact on how SAS programmers work, and explain why validation is such a cornerstone of the programming process in this industry.

1.2 Regulations

There are many layers to the rules and regulations that govern the pharmaceutical industry. As a SAS programmer, you will be required to follow many of these regulations, which can be broken down into three major categories: federal laws, federal guidelines, and industry standards.

Federal laws (the Code of Federal Regulations) consist of legislation that is passed to control how things are done and how information is handled. Violation of these laws can lead to actions such as prosecution by the federal government. Federal guidelines are formal lists of suggestions that the federal government has issued to let the industry know the best way to conduct trials and submit the data in order to enable approval of a drug or device. These guidelines are simply that—guidelines. Unlike laws, failure to follow these guidelines does not carry as hefty a penalty, although it can lead the government to refuse to review a submission or approve a drug. Finally, with time and experience, companies have developed sets of standards that allow information and data to be shared more effectively. As the need for these industry standards has been recognized, organizations have been formed to determine the areas that need standards, to develop suitable standards, and to then document them to share information across companies.

The main source of information on industry standards and requirements is the Food and Drug Administration (FDA). Through various communication channels (primarily regulations and guidance documents published on the agency's Web site, www.fda.gov), the FDA defines the requirements and expectations for a New Drug Application (NDA). While many of the guidance documents and regulations that the FDA issues do not directly impact a SAS programmer's work, some do. Those most relevant to you are discussed here.

1.2.1 Health Insurance Portability and Accountability Act

As summarized by the U.S. Department of Labor (www.dol.gov/dol/topic/health-plans/portability.htm), The Health Insurance Portability and Accountability Act of 1996 (HIPAA)

... provides rights and protections for participants and beneficiaries in group health plans. HIPAA includes protections for coverage under group health plans that limit exclusions for preexisting conditions; prohibit discrimination against employees and dependents based on their health status; and allow a special opportunity to enroll in a new plan to individuals in certain circumstances. HIPAA may also give you a right to purchase individual coverage if you have no group health plan coverage available, and have exhausted COBRA or other continuation coverage.

How does this impact you as a SAS programmer? It has little or no impact on day-to-day programming, but it is important to understand that the law exists and to have a general idea of its purpose. In simple terms, HIPAA serves to protect the information about a subject's identifying information. While this concept has only recently been so plainly articulated, it is the core reason that the most specific identifying information about each subject in every clinical trial conducted in the United States is limited to the subject's initials and date of birth. Any identifying information that is more specific is carefully protected by the investigating site. When validating data that may come to you as a programmer, it is important to understand that personal information should not be included—and if it is, it is your responsibility to point it out to have it removed.

1.2.2 The Code of Federal Regulations

Title 21 of the Code of Federal Regulations (CFR) pertains to food and drugs. Chapter 1 pertains to those components that identify the Food and Drug Administration (FDA) and the Department of Health and Human Services (DHHS). Within this set of regulations, Part 11, perhaps the most well-known and referenced section, specifically identifies electronic records and electronic signatures. It is important to note that any requirements listed under Title 21 in general are often referred to as *predicate rules*.[1] These rules can help determine when Part 11 rules apply to a specific situation, as well as how any aspect of a clinical trial is performed. On the subject of good clinical practice, 21 CFR 50, "Protection of Human Subjects," is one such predicate rule that requires clinical trial subjects to provide written informed consent to participate in a research trial. More indirectly, Part 820.70(i) addresses automated processes: "When computers or automated data processing systems are used as part of production or the quality system, the manufacturer shall validate computer software for its intended use according to an established protocol."[2] While this regulation directly applies to manufacturing, it is the predicate rule that is cited as the reason that SAS programs need to be validated. There are numerous topics within Title 21 that directly (Part 11 and Part 820) or indirectly (Part 50) affect programming. While you don't need to read each of these, it is helpful to understand what parts of the clinical trial and programming process are driven by these rules.

---

[1] www.labcompliance.com/info/links/fda/regulations.aspx
[2] Code of Federal Regulations, Title 21, Volume 8; cite 21CFR820.70

Part 11 of this code contains several sections. Each section outlines the steps to take to ensure that the electronic records, electronic signatures, and handwritten signatures that are applied to electronic clinical data are truthful, dependable, and equal to paper records and handwritten signatures on paper. Most of these regulations are implemented and completed by IT professionals (those responsible for hardware and software installation, documentation, and maintenance). Most important to SAS programmers is the section that dictates how records can be modified: "Use of secure, computer-generated time-stamped audit trails to independently record the date and time of operator entries and actions that create, modify, or delete electronic records. Record changes shall not obscure previously recorded information."[3] The key principal of this regulation is to understand that data cannot just be changed; a specific procedure must be followed. This regulation is the reason that programmers are not permitted to hard code data changes and why a key part of the validation process is ensuring that the result of a programming effort accurately represents the original data that it is based on.

While the FDA has narrowed the scope and application of this regulation, this does not mean that you can disregard these procedures while conducting clinical trials. The FDA is incorporating the general guidelines in this regulation into other regulations and guidance documents, specifically in the Guidance For Industry, Part 11, Electronic Records; Electronic Signatures—Scope and Application. In this document, the FDA clarifies that it has moved to a risk-based approach to this regulation. In it, the FDA "… recommend[s] that you base your approach [to validation] on a justified and documented risk assessment and a determination of the potential of the system to affect product quality and safety, and record integrity." While most SAS programming in the pharmaceutical industry would be considered individual programs rather than systems, the general approach to all programs and the development of relevant standard operating procedures (SOPs) governing validation of those programs should take into account the FDA's thinking on computerized systems.

1.2.3 Guidance for Industry

A series of guidance documents published by the FDA details how information from clinical trials should be submitted. One example of an older guidance document specifically pertaining to programming is *Providing Regulatory Submissions in Electronic Format— General Considerations*.[4] This guidance document provides some detail on how data sets should be structured and which file formats are acceptable. More recently, the FDA has encouraged use of electronic common technical documents (eCTDs) for submissions. See *Providing Regulatory Submissions in Electronic Format— Human Pharmaceutical Product Applications and Related Submissions Using the eCTD Specifications*.[5] This document references a separate guidance that is very relevant for programmers, titled "Study

---

[3] Federal Register, 21 CFR Part 11 – Subpart B §11.10 (e)

[4] www.fda.gov/cber/gdlns/elecgen.htm

[5] www.fda.gov/cder/guidance/7087rev.htm

Data Specifications."[6] As requirements change, the FDA issues these documents to notify the industry of what those changes are and how to comply with them.

For example, currently the FDA accepts data only as SAS Version 5 compatible transport files. This can be challenging at times because most companies now use SAS Version 8 or later. These versions offer much more flexibility and greater functionality than SAS Version 5; specifically, variable names can be longer than 8 characters, character variables can be larger than 200 bytes, and variable labels can be longer than 40 characters. However, due to SAS Version 5 compatibility restrictions, many of these data set features cannot be used. Until this restriction changes, programmers need to remain aware and work with data set structures prior to SAS Version 8 throughout the programming process so significant restructuring of data is not required later.

Another technical issue is the file size restrictions imposed by the FDA. At one time, the maximum file size allowed in a submission was 5 MB. Currently, the maximum file size is 100 MB, and while this may seem adequate for most types of data, keep this restriction in mind when designing all data sets. Unnecessary variables and duplication of information can push the limits of this restriction and cause future issues. While requirements may change over time, it is important to keep abreast of any such issues that could impact how you structure your programs and the output they create.

1.2.4 International Conference on Harmonisation of Technical Requirements

While the US FDA is the world's leading drug approval agency, other countries also develop drugs and have agencies that regulate their approval. In a global setting, it is important for all parties involved in drug development to have a standard set of definitions for similar concepts and a common understanding for how drugs should be developed. This way, companies that develop drugs in one country under one set of rules can apply to have the same drug approved in other countries without having to redevelop it. If all countries have the same understanding of the rules, data developed elsewhere will follow a consistent set of rules. The International Conference on Harmonisation of Technical Requirements for Registration of Pharmaceuticals for Human Use (ICH) is a global organization that provides these common definitions and guidelines and is often a source for standard values for certain data (e.g., *country of origin*). *E6 Good Clinical Practice: Consolidated Guidance*[7] is one of the more general guidance documents published by ICH that defines many common terms (such as adverse drug reaction) and general guidance for how trials should be conducted (such as how safety data should be reported). *E9 Statistical Principles for Clinical Trials*[8] is a more narrow guidance that lays forth

---

[6] www.fda.gov/cder/regulatory/ersr/Studydata.pdf
[7] www.fda.gov/cder/guidance/959fnl.pdf
[8] www.fda.gov/Cder/guidance/ICH_E9-fnl.pdf

the general statistical principles that guide the development of complete programs (what types of studies should be conducted to support claims of safety and efficacy) and how individual studies should be designed (sample size, parallel group or crossover or other design, randomization/blinding, for example) and reported. While these guidance documents may not impact your programming responsibilities directly, they are part of the framework that built the studies and the specifications you work with regularly.

1.2.5 Clinical Data Interchange Standards Consortium

The Clinical Data Interchange Standards Consortium (CDISC) is a team of industry professionals, including members from the FDA. According to CDISC (www.cdisc.org), its mission is "to develop and support global, platform-independent data standards that enable information system interoperability to improve medical research and related areas of healthcare."

In other words, the CDISC end product is a set of data standards that companies in the industry can follow to expedite filing a clinical trials outcome. Each module that CDISC delivers contains the structure, derivation rules, attributes, and components of the data that the FDA will receive. The goal is to achieve a standard set of data that the FDA needs to program only once. Consequent receipt of clinical data can then be analyzed using standard programming, and the review process can be expedited.

It is important for programmers to understand CDISC standards and to realize that CDISC actually has several standards. Two key sets of standards that affect the majority of clinical trial programmers are the Study Data Tabulation Model (SDTM) used for submitting data tabulations and the Analysis Data Set Model (ADaM) used for submitting analysis data sets. While these two sets of standards overlap in many areas, both have many distinct components that can effect how data is stored. Other standards are currently under development, so it is important to keep abreast of the most recent documentation.

While these standards are not yet a requirement, but rather a guideline, the FDA does recommend following them. Ultimately, the use of these standards will depend on your company's policies. These standards are quickly becoming industry standards, so implementing them is highly recommended. Regardless, having a set of standards for data collection and storage such as those provided by CDISC streamlines programming for the pharmaceutical company and expedites the review and approval process for the FDA. Once the CDISC standards have been completed, the FDA will probably adopt them as a requirement for submitting data. Getting to know the CDISC standards now and implementing those standards as much as possible will save time in the future.

1.3 Documentation

Another way that FDA requirements directly affect a SAS programmer's daily responsibilities is in the area of documentation. The term *documentation* refers to several things—both information that programmers work with and information that programmers provide. It can refer to the documents that are used to form the programming structures and ideologies within a company, including standard forms, guidelines, standard operating procedures, and other written guidance documents. It can also mean keeping hardcopy and electronic records of the process and results of programming. In addition, documentation can refer to keeping detailed flow information within a program itself to instruct other users of the purpose and methods used within the program.

All aspects of programming must be documented in one way or another. Documentation is an integral part of the programming process and provides the evidence that your programming efforts were effective. The documentation that is directly involved in programmers' day-to-day activities is discussed in detail in a later chapter. The documentation that is standard for the industry and forms the framework for how programmers perform their job functions, including the requirements for validation, is discussed below.

1.4 Standard Operating Procedures

One key set of documents required by the FDA is standard operating procedures (SOPs). SOPs are documents that describe procedures to follow for a specific operation or task. They detail all aspects of working in the pharmaceutical industry from high-level SOPs (such as defining the process for creating and/or modifying SOPs) to lower-level SOPs (such as defining each step to be followed while programming, validating, and delivering SAS programming output). SOPs may be created for several different levels of clinical trial programs.

In general, if a process is listed or mentioned in the CFR, then there will be an SOP that outlines the process. While following these CFR-related SOPs is required, following other procedures outlined in SOPs (as opposed to guidelines or no guidance at all) is up to the individual company. It is important for programmers to know which SOPs directly influence how their jobs are performed. There are several categories of SOPs that can affect programming processes.

1.4.1 Companywide Standard Operating Procedures

Each pharmaceutical company or clinical research organization (CRO) creates and maintains standard operating procedures for the daily functioning of its business. These high-level SOPs usually contain general company operating guidelines followed by every employee. Typically, they identify:

- company operating structure

- document handling

- employee training

- physical business information

1.4.2 Department Standard Operating Procedures

Each pharmaceutical company or CRO also creates and maintains standard operating procedures for the daily functioning of its individual departments. Programmers are trained in these detailed SOPs, which typically identify:

- using SAS programming standards or guidelines

- computer system structure, usage, and permissions

- randomization scheduling and programming

- blinding and unblinding procedures

1.4.3 Task Standard Operating Procedures

Sometimes programmers must perform job tasks that need to be described in more detail than company and department standard operating procedures. In most cases, a SAS programming department creates task-level SOPs to outline standard procedures for dealing with these varying tasks. Task-level SOPs normally identify procedures to follow to accomplish programming in the following areas:

- importing data

- validating derived or analysis data

- validating summary tables and figures

- exporting of data and/or reports

- studying drug compliance

Each company's SOPs structure and layout may differ, but they all accomplish the same task: creating a standard, structured, and controlled set of procedures for all employees to follow. These standards ensure that tasks are completed consistently and with a similar level of quality. SOPs often specify checklists that include the individual processes that need to be followed to ensure a consistent level of quality. For example, an SOP that details how the validation of data set programs is performed may also have a checklist to be completed for every program that creates a data set. That checklist may include items such as:

- ensure all variables detailed in the specification are included in the data set

- ensure that numeric variables are rounded correctly and per specification

- ensure that values in character variables are not truncated

- check a sample of derived variable values against source data to ensure correct derivation

It is important to know whether your company has SOPs governing validation and what these SOPs include. If they are available, following validation SOPs will help to ensure that each programmer produces the same quality of output.

1.5 SAS Programming Guidelines

Standard operating procedures are normally written as an overview or on a very general level. This generality avoids the need to change the SOPs frequently, when minor details need to change. Because SOPs must be approved by several levels of management and controlled through a document management system, frequent changes become time-consuming and problematic. To avoid making multiple changes to the programming SOPs, SAS programming guidelines are created. These guidelines serve as a more detailed set of instructions for programmers to follow to maintain a consistent program structure and methodology for performing common tasks. The guidelines often outline program structure (headings, comments, white space, and compute blocking, for example), standard calculation formulas, methods for validation, and how to handle deviations from the SOPs. Programming guidelines are often the key to providing consistency between members of a programming team.

Because programming guidelines are not as tightly controlled as SOPs, they allow for more flexibility and change. When a version of SAS changes, operating systems change, or other changes are made, the guidelines can easily be updated, distributed, and taught.

1.6 Quality Control versus Quality Assurance

Quality control (QC) and quality assurance (QA) are important parts of a clinical trials environment. They act to maintain standards and excellence in completing a successful trial. Quality control is defined as "an aggregate of activities (as design analysis and inspection for defects) designed to ensure adequate quality especially in manufactured products."[9] Quality assurance is defined as "a program for the systematic monitoring and evaluation of the various aspects of a project, service, or facility to ensure that standards of quality are being met."[10]

The main difference between QA and QC is that QC is performed within each department. For programmers, QC is maintained using standards and documentation (for example, standard operating procedures and SAS programming guidelines). QC occurs when a programmer checks his or her own output (for example, printing observations from a data set before and after manipulation and then comparing the results) and when two programmers within the same department independently produce output and then compare the results.

On the other hand, QA is performed by an independent group outside of the programming department. In the pharmaceutical industry, this is typically the Regulatory Department. In some companies, this department also has SAS programmers who independently try to replicate the results produced by the programmers in other departments. The Regulatory Department is well-versed in the requirements of both FDA and federal law and will scrutinize all of the clinical trial's output that comes from the company to make sure it is in compliance with these requirements.

1.7 Patient versus Subject

For as long as the industry has been thriving, there has been an ongoing debate about what terminology to use to refer to the participants of clinical trials. In the beginning, the term *patient* was used. As clinical trials became more involved and started going through developmental cycles, the term *subject* was used because many of the trials were being conducted on healthy participants. For consistency, we use the term *subject* to refer to all participants in clinical trials throughout this book.

1.8 Conclusion

There are many rules, regulations, and guidelines that affect a programmer's work and govern the validation process. It is helpful to understand the source of these rules so that any changes are easier to follow. Often these rules can be subject to interpretation. When you are making validation policy decisions, it can be important to refer to the original documentation rather than relying on secondary sources. Detailed sources of information are available for many of the topics discussed in this chapter. Refer to the References section for details. Now that the basis for validation has been established, we can discuss more specific topics that directly influence SAS programming.

---

[9] www.m-w.com/dictionary/quality%20control (Merriam-Webster's Online Dictionary)
[10] www.m-w.com/dictionary/quality%20assurance (Merriam-Webster's Online Dictionary)

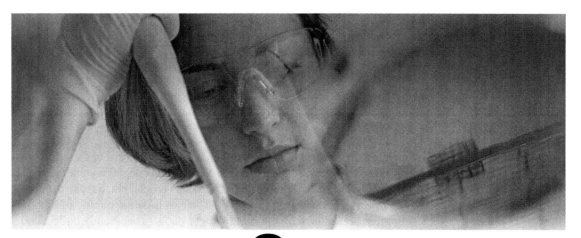

C h a p t e r 2

Validation Overview

2.1 Introduction

Now that we have covered the general need for validation, it is time to discuss validation directly as it applies to the programming process. Validation is necessary not only
because the FDA requires it, but because reporting accuracy is crucial since these data
represent patients or subjects (in other words, people). Their well-being, quality of life
and, above all, safety are represented and reported by these data. To accurately collect and
display clinical study data, the data must undergo rigorous testing and analysis. This process ensures the accuracy and integrity of the measuring device (for example, Case Report Form, clinical database, laboratory data) and the resulting data. This chapter provides
an overview of the general concepts key to performing validation successfully, and later
chapters detail many of the techniques available in SAS to help with this important task.

2.2 Validation versus Verification

Validation is defined as "an act, process or instance of determining the degree of well-
groundedness or justifiability: being at once relevant and meaningful. . . ."[1] *Verification*
is defined as "an act, process or instance of establishing the truth, accuracy, or reality
of. . . ."[2]

The terms are often used synonymously. Validation, a much more in-depth process, is the
act of *proving* that the outcome of a program accurately and effectively represents the
original clinical study data. This takes on many forms and involves a number of procedures, as will be discussed throughout this book. The verification process, a more cursory
review, can take the form of reviewing programming code, reviewing the system through
which the data were collected, and testing the system flow for timeliness and accuracy,
for example. The difference between the two can be defined as follows: Verification is a
confirmation of the system and the data accuracy; validation is a *justification* of the means
used to accomplish the outcome of the program and its accurate representation of the
original data. This justification requires more effort and granular detail to prove that the
data manipulation and analyses were performed correctly and appropriately.

---

[1] www.m-w.com/cgi-bin/dictionary?book=Dictionary&va=valid (Merriam-Webster's Online Dictionary)

[2] www.m-w.com/cgi-bin/dictionary?book=Dictionary&va=verified (Merriam-Webster's Online Dictionary)

The difference between validation and verification is often easier to explain using an example. Assume that weight is collected, either in pounds or kilograms, for each subject in a study. In order to compare weights, any values reported in pounds must be converted to kilograms. The following line of code is included in a DATA step:

```
if unit='lbs' then nweight= round(weight*.4536, .1);
```

Verification entails checking that a given weight run through this formula gives the correct result, perhaps by comparing the SAS result to the result gained by manually performing the calculation on a calculator. In contrast, validation goes a step farther in ensuring that the formula is actually correct and reasonable to use in the given circumstances.

2.3 Why Is Validation Needed?

The most compelling reason to implement and maintain a rigorous validation plan is that validation is an FDA requirement (see 21 CFR Part 820.70(i) and other guidance documents referenced in Chapter 1). During an FDA audit, the auditors review all of the data manipulation and reporting processes. There are, however, several other reasons for validation.

2.3.1 Presenting Correct Information

Important decisions on subject health care are made based on the output generated by programmers. If incorrect information is presented as fact, people's lives could be at risk. It is essential that all data from a clinical trial is presented as accurately as possible so that decisions can be made appropriately. While there is constant pressure in the industry to produce output faster, if that output is incorrect, it could be worse than useless—it could actually be harmful. Careful, diligent validation is the best way to detect and prevent errors.

2.3.2 Validating Early Saves Time

If you validate your work before passing it along, the chance for errors in the final output is much less. Finding errors early and correcting them while you're still familiar with the program is more efficient than finding errors a week later. At that point, the person looking at your output has spent time researching the problem (is it *really* a problem or just misinterpretation?). If the error really is a problem, you need to find the error and fix it. Assuming that the code is documented extensively, this may not take much time, but it will take longer than when the code was originally developed. While it may take a little more time to validate code as you go, it will save significant time later in the process. In an industry where time is money, saving time is a big incentive.

2.3.3 Developing a Positive Relationship

Consistently delivering a quality product to clients is another way that validation helps to develop a positive relationship, which can actually speed the drug development process. A programmer's client may be internal (a statistician, medical writer, or even another programmer) or external (a sponsor, the FDA, or another organization). Without a rigorous validation process, a programmer's work might, and often does, include mistakes (yes, we are human after all). Too many mistakes over time undermine your client's faith in the quality of your work. Without a basic faith in the quality of the output, a reviewer begins to second-guess everything he or she sees. This could lead to a longer review time, a weakening in the relationship with your client, and, at times, a loss of future work.

2.4 How Do You Approach Validation?

One key aspect for approaching the concept of validation is the programmer's attitude. If you approach validation as an unpleasant task, you're not going to be as successful as you need to be. As a programmer, you're the detective looking for evidence that anything is out of place. Not only are you responsible for ensuring that the syntax in the code is correct, you are also responsible for making sure the data meet the assumptions made in the specifications your code is executing. If you're not actively engaged in looking for issues, you will rarely find them. Often it is these overlooked items that wreak havoc with and reduce the quality of output.

Another important aspect to keep in mind during programming is that it is not enough just to *say* you validated a program—you need to have *proof*. Chapter 3 details the documentation that should be used during the process of validation to provide this proof. Depending on the company for which you work, this documentation can vary and serve a variety of purposes. In some cases, it can be used to map out the programming process and convey output discrepancies between programmers, as well as provide proof of validation. The most important thing to keep in mind is that validation and documentation of that validation are requirements.

Chapter 4 begins a discussion of the actual means by which to validate SAS code and the output it produces. But before programming begins, how do you even approach validation? Where do you start? What do you need to effectively and efficiently complete programming and validation?

2.4.1 Start with All the Information

All programmers should start by becoming familiar with the programming specifications. These specifications are very detailed instructions on such issues as the origin of the data, the derivation rules and formulas, and ways to handle problem data. These specifications are typically written by a senior-level programmer or a statistician on a project.

If you work as a programmer in a group that doesn't create programming specifications, create them yourself. Initially it sounds as though this approach might involve more time. In fact, it will save time. If there are no specifications, how can anyone be sure that the code is doing what it is supposed to do? Programming from specifications is much more accurate and efficient than creating rules and standards from moment to moment. Solid specifications enable programmers to validate not only their own work but the work of others when required.

In addition to programming specifications, be sure to obtain all other pertinent documentation. This might include, but is not limited to, Case Report Forms (CRFs), Statistical Analysis Plans (SAPs), Protocols, Protocol Amendments, meeting minutes, and correspondence. All of these documents will aid in the programming and validation efforts for a clinical trial and are detailed in the next chapter.

2.4.2 Have a Plan

It is critical to have a plan before you begin any task in programming. A detailed plan is not necessary at this point; general guidelines are sufficient. Often it's as simple as being clear about the task you need to perform (for example, create a summary table), gathering all of the sources of information you'll need to perform it (annotated CRF, SAP, and so on), understanding the time frame you have to complete the task (needed by Friday), and then starting to program. In many circumstances, the ultimate task (creating the summary table) requires that other tasks are completed first. For example, if you're assigned to create the medical history summary table, you may need to ask if you should create both the analysis data set and/or the data listing that accompanies it. In this case, having a game plan also includes deciding what to do first—the data set would need to come first, but do you need to wait for it to be validated before beginning the table or listing programs? Do you start with the summary table or skip to the table and program the data listing first? In almost all situations, start programming the data listing *before* programming the table. Unless timelines prohibit it, programming data listings before programming summary tables gives you one more chance to look at the data, understand how they work, and identify any issues in the data that could effect how your summary tables perform. This helps not only to validate the analysis data set but the original data that went into it as well. Regardless of the task, taking a few minutes in the beginning to make sure you know where you're going and roughly what needs to be done to get there will ultimately benefit everyone.

2.4.3 Make the Code Do the Work

With all of the time pressures in this industry, it is very important to be efficient with validation techniques. One of the best ways to be efficient is to make the program itself do as much of the checking for you as possible. Because most programs are developed early in the life of the clinical trial database, often "dirty" data is used to test the programs. This data will often have issues such as inconsistent data (height is reported as 200 inches while weight is reported as 65 pounds) and missing data. If the calculations in your program assume that data exists or that it is consistent, programming "data traps" in your code to print any cases that do not meet your assumptions is often helpful. By printing the handful of cases that you know to be a problem, you save time in hunting down problems with output that resulted when the original assumptions were not met. In Chapter 4, we'll discuss how to make your programs do more of the validation work for you.

2.4.4 Ask Questions

As you gain experience in this industry, you tend to ask more questions. By working with different clients, studies, and indications, you'll learn that every clinical trial has its own nuisances and every sponsor has their own preferred way of handling data and analyses. You can't assume that lab data, for example, will be handled in the same way for two different studies. If you find that you need to interpret the specifications, if there is an odd occurrence in the data that was not expected or planned for, or if you have the slightest question about how to approach a problem—**ask someone**. Project team members are happier when you ask questions instead of making an incorrect assumption that results in incorrect output. The fastest way to get your code through validation by peers and/or project team review is to ensure that you understand all of the specifications so you can program accurately the first time.

2.4.5 Be Proactive

Don't wait until the day before a task is due to ask for help or more time. It is not unusual for project team members who are not programmers to make timeline assumptions for programming tasks. This can sometimes lead to unrealistic expectations. For example, you are given two days to program a summary table, which sounds reasonable until you realize that the underlying analysis data set needs to be programmed and validated as well, which could easily take two days alone. In this type of situation, speak with your project manager to either get help or more time. Help doesn't always need to come from other programmers. You may need to think outside the box if time *and* resources are in short supply. For example, often data managers or data entry personnel will have more time when you're the busiest—see if they can help validate data listings. If there are particularly complex data sets or tables to program, ask the statistician for help in validating them. The earlier you realize that you may not have time to program and/or validate a product, the better chance you have to find help to get it done.

In order to know when help is needed, it is important to have a reasonable idea of how long each task will take. The time required to perform a given task will vary based on the company's system (is everything programmed from scratch or are there extensive macro programs that can speed the process?) and the extent and quality of the specifications you're working from (high-level specifications with little detail or very well-thought-out, detailed specifications). For example, programming a summary table of subject demographics (age, sex, race, ethnicity) may take four hours to program from scratch, two hours if there are similar programs from other studies to borrow from, or only half an hour if there is a standard table macro that can simply be called with the appropriate parameters. In general, data sets take the longest amount of time to program, tables and figures are a close second, and listings take the least amount of time. Keep track of how long tasks take to complete in order to get an accurate feel for how long new, similar tasks will take in the future. If you aren't sure how long a given task is expected to take, ask a project manager or other senior programmer for their thoughts. This way, you can better gauge when time will run out and know when it's time to ask for help.

2.4.6 Validation Must Come First

Cutting corners in this industry only ends up costing more in the long run. There will always be time pressures at some point in the clinical trial process—data may not be collected as quickly as expected and programmers are expected to help make up some of the lost time; the people responsible for generating the timelines didn't have a good understanding of how long programming tasks take; unexpected changes in the analyses occurred that were not accounted for in the original timelines; insufficient programming resources are available to produce the output in the time allotted. These are among any number of reasons why you are now crunched for programming time. Regardless of the reasons for a shortened timeline, validation should always be your primary concern. Never let yourself be pressured into handing over work as complete unless the output has been validated. The best way to shorten the process without sacrificing quality is to let your programs do most of the work for you. In the rest of this chapter and in following chapters, we discuss not only how to approach tasks but how to approach them intelligently so that the programs do most of the work.

2.5 Validation Methods

There are generally two ways to approach validation of output: separate, independent programming and peer review. Each method has its strengths and weaknesses, and there is no single correct approach. Every company evaluates these methods and chooses one or the other. Rarely are both methods used for validation; in some cases, independent programming is used to validate output, while peer review is used as a training tool for new or junior programmers.

2.5.1 Independent Programming

Independent programming involves using two different programmers to program output and then comparing the finished results. The two steps involved in this type of validation programming are often referred to as *first-level validation* and *second-level validation*. Depending on where you work, you may find these two concepts referred to with different terminology (such as first-round and second-round validation or production validation and QC validation). Regardless of the terms, the concepts are the same.

2.5.1.1 First-Level Validation

First-level validation is performed by a programmer during development of the original (production) programming suite; this is a group of programs that manipulate data, perform the data analysis, and create the tables/listings/figures (TLFs). The output of these programs will be delivered to people outside of the programming group for use in generating the Clinical Study Report. All of the programming completed during the beginning of a study is considered to be in development. During this time, programs may be altered many times. While validation should be completed after each alteration of a program, it is not considered final until the program is complete and sent to an independent validation programmer.

First-level validation is often glossed over by programmers due to time pressure and the expectation that the validator will uncover any issues. Many programmers do not verify that each step in the program is correct as it is being programmed. Unfortunately, skipping this vital piece of the process actually lengthens the programming in the end. If you are responsible for creating production programs, remember that validation of your own program is just as important as producing output.

2.5.1.2 Second-Level Validation

Second-level validation is performed by a programmer who did not write the original programming code to create the output. This programmer writes these programs independently from the original programmer. The goal of this programming effort is to produce the same output as the first-level validation without knowledge of the means used by the original programmer. Often an analysis is common and the same means to an end may be used. The important element to remember is that validation programming is separate and *independent* from the original. Should there be a question or issue about the programming, check with a senior-level person (perhaps the programming project leader or the statistician for the project). The second-level validator should not ask questions of the original programmer. This can introduce bias into the programming and invalidate the independence. This is a key concept for a number of reasons.

The differences between original and validation program results are rarely due to syntax errors or incorrect use of the SAS language. The most common cause of discrepancies is different interpretations of the specifications provided. One programmer may have missed reading a table footnote that impacted how a value should be calculated. Perhaps the specifications were not completely clear and thus left room for interpretation, and each programmer interpreted differently. Sometimes the data were not collected exactly as originally anticipated, the specifications did not take these new variations into account, and each programmer handled the new data differently.

Probably the second most common cause of output difference is related to data issues that become apparent when two programmers approach the same problem with two different methods (there are at least two ways, usually more, to approach any given problem in SAS). Often it's not that either program is incorrect, it's that the data is inconsistent with the original database specification (for example, the database specs say that the SPECIFY field should be filled in only if RACE is OTHER; however, there is a case where RACE is WHITE, but the SPECIFY field is still filled in). In cases where discrepancies are found to be caused by data inconsistencies (if the problem in the data gets fixed, both programs will produce the same result), it is important to check with the data management team to find out whether or not that data inconsistency will be fixed. If the database will be updated to fix the issue, both the first- and second-level programmers usually leave their code as it is, and then they check the results again once the data have been finalized to ensure that the issue was resolved. If the data will not be updated to resolve the inconsistency, whoever wrote the specifications for the output may need to provide additional details on how to handle the data inconsistency causing the programs to disagree.

The following items describe the strengths and weaknesses of this method:

- Strengths: Catches errors in spec interpretation, SAS logic errors; can reproduce easily if new data; allows for junior-level programmers to work effectively in the production or validation environment.

- Weaknesses: Time-consuming/expensive; only catches errors after the code has been executed.

2.5.2 Peer Review

Validation using peer review involves only one programmer creating programs. As with independent programming, the programmer responsible for creating the production code is responsible for ensuring that the output of that code is correct; they must validate their own code first. Once the program that generates output is complete, the code is then reviewed by another programmer. This is the main difference between independent programming, where a second program is created and only the final output is reviewed. In general, the more senior programmer reviews the code side by side with the specification and verifies that they match. Often the log from the program is also reviewed to make sure that there were no syntax errors and that the number of observations makes sense from DATA step to DATA step. For TLFs, peer review may also involve reviewing the final output to ensure that the layout matches the specification and cross-checking between related output to ensure that the results are consistent (for example, ensuring that the counts in the table match the number of records in the corresponding listing).

The following items describe the strengths and weaknesses of this method:

- Strengths: Fast; can catch logic errors prior to final execution of the code.

- Weaknesses: If anything changes, need to redo; can miss syntax issues and issues with interpretation of specifications; really need senior staff on the validation side to do this effectively.

2.6 Validation Checklists

Given the number and variety of items that programmers are responsible for validating, it is often helpful to have a list of items that need to be checked. It is fairly common for companies to have such checklists available, either as part of their SOPs or as guideline documents. These checklists are often grouped by task; items to check when creating analysis data sets can differ from the items to check when creating summary tables or figures. Appendix A contains several examples of validation checklists. Regardless of the task being performed, it is possible to detail items that should be checked across almost any task:

- Clean logs—There should never be any warnings or errors in the program log.

- Adequate, accurate documentation—Is there a program header? Is there enough documentation within the code to easily find the major sections of logic? Do the comments in the code accurately describe what the code is doing?

- Output looks like the specification—For TLFs, does the layout match the specification? Are all words in the titles and footnotes spelled correctly?

- Output content matches the specification—Did the result of the program match what the specification required?

- Output content matches similar content on other output—If other output reports the same information as the current output, do they match?

- Output content makes sense—Even if the program performed exactly as the-specification required, does the output make logical sense given the data that is available? Does the specification need to be reviewed in light of unexpected data?

This validation list outlines the basic requirements with which to begin. This list will grow as different tasks and types of data are discussed.

2.7 Software Development Life Cycle

In any area where programming is used, whether it is programming in SAS or in Visual Basic, the software development life cycle (SDLC) is part of the process. The main difference is how formally that development cycle is outlined, documented, and followed. In most cases, when the SDLC is referenced, it implies that there is a formal process that is followed and documented from the start of the programming process through to final code development and maintenance. While many different SDLC models are available, the most commonly used involve the following phases: requirements, design, implementation, testing (validation), and maintenance.[3][4][5] In the requirements phase, programmers meet with the client to determine exactly what the client wants the program to do. During the design phase, programmers design on paper exactly how the program will accomplish those requirements. The code is actually written based on the design plan during the implementation phase. Testing validates that the final product met the requirements. Once the finished product is released to the client, any changes are executed and documented in the maintenance phase. Within a formal SDLC process, each phase is thoroughly documented and may have an associated SOP.

Inherent in the name of this process is the word *software*, which, strictly speaking, refers to the programs used to direct the operation of a computer, as well as documentation giving instructions on how to use them.[6][7][8] In practice, most of us think of software as a multi-use package such as Microsoft Word or Internet Explorer and not unique programs that are written to perform one specific function (such as a SAS program that creates a summary table of medical history information reported for a specific study). For the complete software systems required to fulfill a flexible set of requirements (such as MS Word where you can create documents, but each document is unique and built by the user), a formal SDLC process serves to organize the development of the software and thus makes the process more efficient. However, software packages are much larger scale, broader scope endeavors than most programs created for analyzing and summarizing clinical trial

---

[3] www.stylusinc.com/Common/Concerns/SoftwareDevtPhilosophy.php

[4] www.elucidata.com/refs/sdlc.pdf

[5] www.computerworld.com/developmenttopics/development/story/0,10801,71151,00.html

[6] American Psychological Association (APA): software. Dictionary.com Unabridged (v 1.1). Random House, Inc. http://dictionary.reference.com/browse/software.

[7] Chicago Manual Style (CMS): software. Dictionary.com Unabridged (v 1.1). Random House, Inc. http://dictionary.reference.com/browse/software.

[8] Modern Language Association (MLA): software. Dictionary.com Unabridged (v 1.1). Random House, Inc. http://dictionary.reference.com/browse/software.

data. At some point, the benefit provided by extensive documentation at the beginning is not worth the cost involved.

A more formal program development process is beneficial when you are creating macros that are intended for general use. A macro that can convert character dates that are entered in multiple formats into numeric dates and impute partially missing dates as part of the process is an example. This type of macro needs to do several tasks (impute missing data as well as convert formats) across multiple programs (both within a single study and across multiple studies). Because the code is intended for wide use, it needs to meet even more rigorous validation standards. To facilitate this vigorous testing, it is imperative to have clear requirements that state exactly what the code is supposed to do and how. Based on these requirements, a thorough test plan can be developed and implemented to ensure that the code performs as expected. Specific guidance on how any changes are made to the code after it has been approved for use will need to be developed. Changing this code could now potentially affect hundreds of other programs, not just the one the modification is needed for.

For single-use or unique "one-off" programs that have a very specific purpose, often the SAP or data specifications are sufficient to satisfy the requirements phase. The design stage is often not applicable because only one task is being performed (generating a summary table); it does not add to the process to detail when you need to sort data sets and merge them. Implementation occurs and validation is part of both the implementation (the programmer checks the code as it is written) and after the implementation (either a second-level validation or peer review). Maintenance is often a minor task with these types of programs; it does not happen often, and when it does usually only the code in question is affected.

2.8 Conclusion

This chapter has identified validation, its purpose, and why it is required, and provided a brief overview of the documentation needed to accomplish it. Validation is a crucial and required element of programming and can mean everything to the timely delivery of accurate and efficient SAS output. In the next chapter, we focus on how documentation and good programming practices can aid in the process of validation.

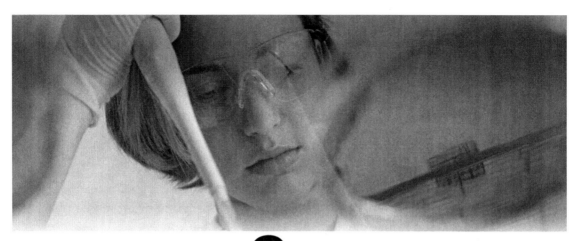

C h a p t e r **3**

Documentation and Maintenance

3.1 Introduction

In the pharmaceutical industry, documentation is an integral part of the validation process. As mentioned previously, the term *documentation* refers to several things: forms, guidelines, SOPs, and other written information; hardcopy and electronic records; and the detailed flow information stored within a program itself. Programmers deal with two major types of documentation—the documentation given to us (various programming specifications) and the documentation created by us (e.g., validation checklists). Often the specifications that programmers work with are scattered across several documents rather than neatly packaged in one comprehensive list. In addition to the documentation given to us, programmers need to provide quite a bit of documentation—again often in many pieces. Documentation of both what a programmer did (and often why) and what a programmer created (and how) are key factors in successful validation in this industry.

Validating the methodology used to produce a result, the data used to produce output, or the final output itself begins with several types of documentation. You need to document the data you'll be using, what will need to be done with it, and, in some cases, how it needs to be done. It is often this documentation that directly influences what is validated and how the validation is done.

In addition to the initial information, often the validation process requires some documentation from the programmer as well—filling out validation checklists or documenting what was done in the program (and possibly why). This type of validation documentation often serves one of two purposes—providing proof that the validation process was followed or providing detail about code or data that may be questioned later. This chapter discusses several types of documentation that may be required as part of the overall validation process.

3.2 Starting the Process

Before programming can begin, a pharmaceutical programmer needs several key documents to effectively complete a programming task. Assembling all of this documentation before programming begins makes the process easier, faster, and more accurate. Programmers need this documentation to make validation possible—without specifications, there is no way to validate. Depending on the task, all or some of the following may be used:

- Study Protocol and amendments

- Annotated Case Report Form (aCRF)

- Statistical Analysis Plan (including programming specifications for analyses and mock-ups)

- Data Set Specifications

- Relevant meeting minutes, e-mails, and other documentation

3.2.1 Study Protocol

The *study protocol* is a detailed description of the clinical study being performed. It is a road map for the investigators, monitors, and other clinicians who conduct and execute the trial. The protocol is created before the clinical trial begins and often changes during the trial when issues and concerns are discovered. Any changes made to the protocol must be completed using an amendment process so that the original document remains intact. As a result, the original protocol does not always contain all the information needed to understand how the data was collected for a trial—the amendments are also required to complete the picture.

You should read the protocol and all amendments before beginning to program. They provide you with the background and purpose of the study and offer insight into aspects of the trial that will influence how programs are constructed and what to review during validation. The timing of events that occur throughout the study, the type of information collected, and general guidelines about how the data will be analyzed are all discussed and explained in the protocol. This information is important in helping you understand the scope of your programming task. While it is not necessary to read the entire document, programmers should review the relevant sections. The statistical and data collection sections could add valuable insight into the original intent of the analysis (what, why, and how). By reading this information, you can gain the broader perspective needed to do true, quality work.

3.2.2 Annotated Case Report Form

The *Case Report Form* (CRF) is the medium through which clinical data is collected. It can either be physical paper pages or electronic "pages" that are completed by the investigator with information from every subject visit over the course of the trial. Most often, the CRF contains the following areas of interest (Note: These types of data are discussed in depth in later chapters):

- Demographics—General subject information, including initials, birth date, gender, and race

- Inclusion criteria—Criteria that a subject must meet to be included in the study

- Exclusion criteria—Criteria that, if met, exclude a subject from the study

- Vital signs—Height, weight, blood pressure, pulse, respiration, and any other vital signs collected

- Medical history—Relevant medical history for the subject collected before the study starts

- Physical exam—A full physical exam of the subject performed before and/or after the first dose of study medication

- Laboratory tests—Hematology, blood chemistry, and urinalysis results before, during, and/or after the study

- Concomitant medications—Any medications in addition to the study medication that the subject takes

- Adverse events—Any untoward or unexpected event that a subject experiences during the study

- Subject compliance—How compliant the subject was in taking his/her study medication

- Disposition—End-of-study information, including the reason the subject is no longer in the trial

- Comments—Any comments recorded by the investigator or designee

An *annotated CRF* (aCRF) is simply a CRF that has been annotated with the variable names (and often type and length) from the database that correspond to the items on the page. The annotated CRF provides a "visual" look at the data in the database and facilitates the programming process. Reviewing the data with the CRF provides an idea of what to expect for variable values and can also give insight into what values make sense between variables (for example, if AGE is 6 years old, you would not expect HEIGHT to be over 6 feet). While most annotated CRFs include only variable names, inclusion of attributes that are typically found in output from PROC CONTENTS (such as variable type and length) can be very helpful. Consider the simplified demographic portion of the CRF in Example 3.1:

Example 3.1

Demographics

Investigator _____   Subject Number _____   Subject Initials _____

Date of Birth: __ __ | __ __ | __ __ __ __

                m   m   d   d   y   y   y   y

Sex at Birth: Male   Female

Race: Caucasian   Black   Asian   Hispanic   American Indian

       Other (specify): _____

The PROC CONTENTS output displays the following information:

Output 3.1

```
Header information...

          Alphabetic List of Variables and Attributes

  # Variable Type Len Format       Informat      Label

  1 BARCODE  Char  25                             Bar Code
 12 BIRTHDT  Num    8 MMDDYY10.    MMDDYY10.    Date of Birth
  7 DATESTMP Num    8 DATETIME17.  DATETIME17.  Date/Time\Stamp
  8 E_STAT   Char   1                             Data Entry\Status
  3 INV_NO   Num    8                             Investigator\Number
  4 PAGENO   Char   8                             Segment
  2 PATID    Num    8                             Patient\I.D.
  5 PROTO    Char  20                             Protocol
 14 RACECD   Num    3                             Race
 15 RACEOTH  Char  30                             Race Specify
  9 SCREENNO Num    4                             Screening Number
  6 SEQ      Num    3                             Sequence\No.
 13 SEXCD    Num    3                             Sex
 10 SUBJINIT Char   3                             Patient Initials
 11 VISIT    Char   6                             Visit
```

Notice that there are many more variables included in the data set than appear on the CRF page itself. Data management system variables are commonly included in data sets. It is important to know what these variables are so they can be included or excluded as appropriate. Example 3.2 shows the annotated CRF using the output from Output 3.1. Note that the demographics data set name would be presented in red ❶ and the variable names and attributes would be presented in green❷. Any electronic annotations should not be in blue because the FDA requirements state that only hyperlinks can be blue.

Example 3.2

Demographics   DEMO ❶

       INV_NO N8. ❷   **PATID N8. ❷**   **SUBJINIT Char3. ❷**

Investigator _____   Subject Number _____   Subject Initials _____

Date of Birth: __ __ | __ __ | __ __ __ __   **BIRTHDT MMDDYY10. ❷**
               m m   d d   y y y y

Sex at Birth: Male   Female   **SEXCD N3. ❷**

Race: Caucasian   Black   Asian   Hispanic   American Indian

       Other (specify): _____   **RACECD N3. ❷**
                                       RACEOTH Char30. ❷

Keep in mind that the annotated CRF is generally created at the beginning of the project, before any data is available for entry. During the course of the trial, information may be provided on the paper CRF that was not accounted for in the database. In some cases, the database may need to be adjusted to capture this information. For example, extra comment fields may allow multiple answers to a given question or different combinations of answers. The annotated CRF is not always a final, static representation of the database. These data changes are one of the key reasons for discrepancies during the validation process. It is important to keep the data itself in mind when assumptions about the data are critical to the logic being programmed.

The annotated CRF always reflects the database as it was entered (the "original" data as programming receives it from data management). It is also becoming more common to see a second annotated CRF that includes the variables as they appear in the data sets that the TLFs are created from (the "submission" or "analysis" data). Sometimes information from the CRF cannot be entered into the database in a structure that is ultimately required for submission to the FDA because of issues with database software and data entry efficiency. In these cases, you need to write programs that reshape the data into a standard format that is both efficient for programming TLFs and acceptable for submission to the FDA. In this process, variable names and types may be changed so that the original annotated CRF no longer reflects the data actually being submitted. Any recipient of this submission data needs an updated submission annotated CRF that reflects what is actually in the database. Programmers are often responsible for helping to create this document. It is important to understand that even though the document itself is not a SAS program, the content must be validated against the SAS data sets the document represents. This involves comparing the document to the content of the data set and ensuring that they match.

3.2.3 Statistical Analysis Plan

The *Statistical Analysis Plan* (SAP) defines the statistical analysis that will be performed for the clinical trial and all of the SAS output required to be included in the Clinical Trial Report (CTR). The SAP and the annotated CRF are the two documents most often used by the programmer to complete the programming assignments required for the trial. The level of detail provided in the SAP can vary, but for the purposes of this book it is assumed to include the following:

- A brief description of the study and its purpose

- The statistical methods to be used—how subject data will be summarized (descriptive statistics such as mean and standard deviation or counts with percents), the statistical tests to be used (Fisher's Exact Test and two-tailed *t*-tests, for example), and so on

- Data-handling rules for reporting purposes—when and how to impute missing/ partial dates, what combination of values qualifies a subject for efficacy analysis, and so on

- A complete table of contents with all TLFs to be programmed

- Mocks (or shells) of all unique TLFs to be programmed—representations of what each TLF will look like but without the actual numbers

Within this context, there are variations on the specific content of the analysis plan. For example, some companies include the study description and statistical methods in one document, the data-handling rules in another document, and the table of contents for the TLFs and mockups in yet another document. These documents as a whole are the core of the specifications needed for programming. Appendix B includes one sample of an abbreviated SAP; a typical table of contents for a SAP is outlined in Example 3.3.

Example 3.3

1. Study Objectives

2. Study Design

3. Study Evaluations

    3.1 Demographic and Baseline Characteristics

    3.2 Efficacy Evaluations

    3.3 Safety Evaluations

4. Statistical Methods and Documentation of Sample Size

    4.1 Statistical and Analytical Plans

        Data Handling

        Demographic and Baseline Characteristics

        Medical History

        Prior and Concomitant Medications

        Extent of Exposure and Compliance

        Efficacy Analysis

        Primary Response Variable

        Secondary Response Variables

        Pharmacokinetic Analysis

        Safety Analysis

        Interim Analysis

    4.2 Determination of Sample Size

    4.3 Changes in the Conduct of the Study or Planned Analysis

5. Statistical Software

Programming Specifications

List of Tables

List of Subject Data Listings

Mockups of Tables and Subject Data Listings

It is important for programmers to read *all* of the analysis plan before programming, not just review the mockups. The study description, methods for analysis, and data-handling rules will often add perspective to individual TLFs. Items you may have reviewed that pertain to other types of data may lead you to raise questions regarding the data with which you are currently working. For example, the SAP often provides data-handling rules about partially missing dates. A programmer who is creating a medical history listing may read rules for dealing with partial dates for the concomitant medication listing. Some medical history findings have partial dates; the programmer can ask the statistician if missing medical history dates should be handled in the same manner as missing concomitant medication dates.

When you are programming, realize that the SAP author assumes that the data in the database will behave exactly as specified in the protocol and CRF completion guidelines. Often this is not the case. As a result, the SAP may not contain all of the rules necessary to handle every idiosyncrasy in the data. It is also important to remember that the people writing the SAP are human and, therefore, capable of making mistakes. Considering the amount of detail that goes into this kind of document, the probability of something being overlooked is high. Never be afraid to question the specifications. Usually the authors appreciate having a second set of eyes review the document so that any oversight is caught early rather than after significant effort has been spent to program. While the SAP may have minor changes over the course of a clinical trial, it is important that this document be kept current. The SAP is the main specification source used both for programming TLFs and validating the results of that programming.

3.2.4 Meeting Minutes

During a trial, items can be missed; unexpected issues can arise in the data collection effort as well as in the data responses themselves. The nature of these issues and the decisions made about handling them are often documented in various meeting minutes, e-mails, memos, and other ad-hoc documentation sources. Ideally, a member of the programming team will be included in regular project team meetings to be aware of any issues that may affect programming. If this is not possible, programmers should have access to these documents. This is particularly critical if a second, independent programmer will be validating your output—if both programmers do not have all of the information pertaining to a task, the validation process will take significantly longer. To maximize opportunities for efficiency, it is essential that programmers be involved throughout the trial process.

3.3 Internal Program Documentation

Probably the most important documentation that programmers create is that in the code itself. Unfortunately, in the press to complete programs quickly, this is often the step that many programmers omit. In the pharmaceutical industry, programs and output are used and/or referenced months and even years after creation. Often, paper documentation gets lost in the archive process while the code itself is more readily accessible. In addition, if programmers are asked how something was calculated, the first place they are comfortable looking is within the program itself. If the program has no comments explaining what's going on (and often why), it will often take much longer to review the code and find the answer. Many times, code is added based on clarification of a specification while the original specification does not get updated. If there is a question regarding the validity of the program output, often a well-placed comment will either answer the question or reference documentation that does. In addition, code is often copied from one study to another and modified as needed rather than starting from scratch. In these cases, the relevance of specific code to the study at hand may come into question—comments can also help answer these questions. The three key program documentation areas include program headers detailing what the program does, comments throughout the code explaining what's going on and why, and titles included with output.

3.3.1 Program Header

The program header appears as the first lines in any program. This should contain general information needed about the program, including the following:

- Program name

- Program author

- General purpose of the program

- Data used

- Output created

- Version of SAS with which the program was created

- The study for which the program was created

- Brief description of changes made to the program after change control was initiated

This list contains the minimum items that should be included in any program used to create analysis data sets and TLFs. Some items, such as the study the program was created for, may not be applicable for some programs, such as general library macros. In addition, some companies may require more information in the header, such as listing any macros that are used. Even if the company for which you work does not have a required program header, you can take the initiative to include the above information at the top of each program.

These items are important because programs are copied and reused across multiple projects. When a programmer is searching for code to reuse, it is often not obvious from the name of the program what that program actually does. If the header includes this information, it is easy to open programs and immediately have the key information needed to decide if the code can be useful.

Of particular interest from a validation standpoint is the program modification information. Once a program has been validated and the output deemed accurate, any changes to the code should be documented in the program header. In this way, if there are differences between output over time (for example, between a draft run and a final run), the reasons for those differences are easy to find. In addition, any discrepancies found by the person validating your output could be explained by these changes as well. Changes documented in the program header can save a significant amount of time in tracking down why differences in any output exist.

Including the version of SAS alerts others using the code of any potential issues involved in running the code. For example, clinical trials can often take several years to complete. If the original programs were created in SAS 6.12 and you are now programming with SAS 9, there will likely be issues when running statistical procedures where data sets are created, because many variable names have changed between the versions. An example of a good program header is provided in Example 3.4.

Example 3.4

```
/*-----------------------------------------------------------------**
** PROGRAM:    LMH.SAS
** CREATED:    02/2005
** PURPOSE:    CREATE MEDICAL HISTORY DATA LISTING
** PROGRAMMER: C. MATTHEWS
** INPUT:      SUBLIB.MH
** OUTPUT:     LMH.LST
** PROTOCOL:   ABC-123
** MODIFIED:   DATE        BY          NOTE
**             --------- ----------- --------------------------
**-----------------------------------------------------------------**
**   PROGRAMMED USING SAS VERSION 8.2                          **
**-----------------------------------------------------------------**/
```

3.3.2 Body Comments

The next important form of internal documentation is the comments included throughout the body of the program (the part of the program after the header that actually does something). Body comments play several key roles throughout the course of a program. First, they visually break conceptual blocks of code into major sections, enabling the programmer to quickly and easily find the section of code that needs modification. The second role of body comments is to explain unusual and/or complex code. A comment explaining what a piece of code is doing and the reasoning behind it can save time when a program needs to be modified later or, if validation is performed via peer review, it can help the reviewer understand what specifications are being addressed in this section of code. Good documentation also enables another programmer to know if the code is appropriate for a new project. Finally, body comments can be used to help document changes made to programs after they were finished. Once a program has been finished and validated, changes should be documented with comments such as when the change was made, who requested it, and why.

While body comments are necessary for a number of reasons, it is possible to overdo this. Putting a comment on every line of code does not add value to the program. In fact, overuse of comments can make the program more difficult to read. It is important to strike a balance and include only useful, valuable comments. An example of good body commenting is provided in Example 3.5.

Example 3.5

```
**-----------------------------------------------------------------**;
**   SUMMARY COUNTS OF EACH DEMOGRAPHIC CHARACTERISTIC BY SITE   **;
**-----------------------------------------------------------------**;
proc sort data=sublib.dm_ex1 (keep=siteid sitesubj sex race)
           out=demo;
   by siteid sitesubj;
run;

data demo;
   set demo (rename=(race=racec));
   by siteid sitesubj;

   length race $30.;
   ** PER SAP, IF RACE IN (HISPANIC, AMERICAN INDIAN) THEN
      REPORT THEM WITH OTHER **;
   if racec not in ('Caucasian' 'Black' 'Asian') then
        race = 'Other';
   else race = trim(left(racec));
```

```
   ** CREATE NUMERIC SORT VARIABLES TO ORDER SEX AND RACE **;
   racen = index('CBAO',substr(race,1,1));
        if sex eq 'M' then sexn = 1;
   else if sex eq 'F' then sexn = 2;

   output;

   ** CREATE RECORD FOR TOTAL ACROSS SITES **;
   siteid = '99';
   output;
run;
```

3.3.3 Output Titles

Last, the titles included in any output generated by the program are also considered a form of documentation and help prove that validation was performed. Another person reviewing the output, even something as simple as output from a PROC PRINT, should not have to guess at what is being presented. Accurate, complete titles in output can save valuable time when reviewing and can also prevent confusion and misinterpretation of results. Even something as simple as "10 obs From Incoming AE Data Set" can avoid confusion. If the OBS= option is set in the PROC PRINT statement, including that fact in the output title prevents confusion about the number of observations actually in the data. It may not be obvious to someone unfamiliar with the data that the AE data set has more than 10 observations.

3.4 External Documentation

In addition to the documentation included within each program, there are requirements for documentation outside of the programs themselves. Most drug development programs continue over several years, and both the data and SAS programs are submitted to regulatory agencies. It is critical that each permanent data set and program be documented so that anyone unfamiliar with the project can navigate efficiently and effectively through the sea of files created for each project. In addition, this documentation provides the evidence that any validation procedures required by SOPs have been followed.

3.4.1 Data Definition Tables

Data definition tables (DDTs) are documents that list a variety of information about data sets. They are essentially PROC CONTENTS documents that detail the structure of each data set and how the values in each variable were obtained or derived. The traditional DDT includes one table for each data set with columns for variable name, description, type, and details about how it was created. For example, in the demography data set, AGE would be detailed as "(STARTDT – BIRTHDT)/365.25 rounded down to the nearest whole number." In many cases, companies include additional information such as the length of character variables and the formatted values of coded variables (for example, 1=Yes, 2=No) with the DDT. There are two philosophies about when these documents should be created—the first dictates that the DDT is created before programming begins; the other, that it be created after programming is finished. Regardless of when this document is created, it is the programmer's responsibility to ensure that, in the end, this document accurately reflects the content of each data set. A sample DDT would look something like Example 3.6.

Example 3.6

DMAD.xpt—Demographics Analysis Data

Variable Name	Variable Label	Type	Comments
STUDYID	Study Identifier	Char	Set to "ABC-123"
SUBJID	Subject Identifier	Char	CRF (all pages)
AGE	Age at Reference Date	Num	(RFSTDT-BRTHDT)/365.25 rounded down to the nearest whole number
BRTHDT	Date of Birth	Num	CRF (page S3)
RFSTDT	Subject Reference Start Date	Num	Date of first dose of study drug (CRF page A1)

3.4.2 Program Directory

In addition to documenting data sets, programmers are also responsible for documenting the programs that are created in the course of creating clinical trial output. This includes programs that create data sets, tables, listings, and figures as well as any stand-alone macros that may support those programs. In many cases, the program directory can be as simple as a table of contents with the program and output filename added. Notice in the example below that the single program LAE.SAS creates two listings.

Example 3.7

Report Number	Report Title	Program (*.sas)	Output file (*.RTF)
Table 1.1	Subject Disposition	TPDISP	T1_1
Table 1.2	Subject Demographics	TDEMO	T1_2
Table 2	Medical History Findings	TMHIST	T2
Listing 1.1	Adverse Events Related to Study Drug	LAE	L1_1
Listing 1.2	Adverse Events Leading to Discontinuation	LAE	L1_2

3.4.3 Validation Files

Validation files can be either electronic, paper, or, most often, some combination of the two. These files can contain the following:

- Production SAS programs (programs that create the final output delivered by programming)

- Validation SAS programs (programs created during second-level validation to validate production programs)

- SAS logs

- Validation output (such as intermediate PROC output from production programs and PROC COMPARE results from validation programs)

- Completed validation checklists

- Any relevant documentation (e-mails and meeting minutes, for example)

- Change control documentation

Programmers need to know their company's standards for validation files (the documentation to include, and the medium—paper or electronic). It is easier and less time-consuming to gather the necessary pieces throughout the process than to wait until the end.

3.5 Make Programs Maintainable

One of the most important aspects of programming in the pharmaceutical industry is making the process faster and easier. Time is usually of the essence when programming and making programs easier to access, understand, modify, maintain, execute, and manage is very important. Due to the nature of the work in this industry, code is often be reused over the course of many years for other projects, often by a different programmer than the one who created it. In addition, programs may need to be adjusted months after they were finished. Questions regarding the validity of the code are quickly and efficiently answered when the code is easy to read, easy to understand, and well-documented. There are several ways to accomplish this.

3.5.1 Create and Follow Naming Conventions

Follow meaningful naming conventions for program names, output filenames, and data set and variable names. Even intermediate data sets and variables should have meaningful names that try to describe the content of the item. Programs are often much longer than the piece of code that is displayed on the screen. It may be difficult to remember what data is stored in VAR1 after several hours and many pages of code. Naming the variable something meaningful like TOTAL_*N* will easily avoid such confusion.

Naming programs and output files is another key aspect to making programs maintainable. Giving programs cryptic names like DS1.SAS, DS2.SAS, and so on is not helpful when looking for a specific program in a directory of over 100 programs. Which program creates the medical history data set—DS2.SAS or DS15.SAS?! Establishing naming conventions that provide a clue to the function of the program saves time finding what is needed. It's like looking in a filing cabinet full of folders—isn't it easier to find the exact file needed when each folder has a descriptive label (rather than simply 1–50)? An example of meaningful program file naming conventions follows: The first letter of the program name indicates what type of task it does (D = data sets, T = tables, L = listings, G = graphs); the second two characters are the data set name (assuming the CDISC data set naming convention of unique, two-letter data set names is used); and the remaining five letters can be used to qualify further if necessary. Using this convention, the program DADAE.SAS creates the adverse event analysis data set ADAE, TAESUM.SAS creates the adverse events summary table, TAEBSYS.SAS creates the adverse events by body system table, and LAE.SAS creates the adverse events listing. Using a naming convention like this helps find the appropriate program when looking in a directory full of files.

3.5.2 Make It Easy to Read

All programmers eventually develop their own style of programming—how they structure the code on the page as well as which techniques they use to accomplish a task. In this industry perhaps more than any other, how the code is structured on the page is almost as important as what it is doing. Some key elements that should be considered when writing code are discussed here. Keep in mind that while the examples presented are simple, the impact of the suggestions made is much greater as the programs get longer and more complex. Getting in the habit of structuring code well for all programs (simple and complex) makes it less of a chore when it's really important. Debugging code is difficult enough without struggling to read it.

3.5.2.1 One Statement per Line

The simplest way to make code easy to read is to put no more than one SAS statement per line. It's fine for a long statement to span several lines, but don't program a paragraph. Keeping code spread out helps in a number of ways. First and foremost, the code is easier to debug. Missing semicolons, unmatched quotation marks, and unclosed do-loops are just some of the places where jumbled code makes finding the errors more difficult. Programming one statement per line also makes it easier to follow logic and visually read what the code is doing. When reading lines that do not span the page, the brain naturally pauses at the end of the line. If the end of the line is the end of the statement, you can process the code more efficiently while looking at it. Consider the following example.

Example 3.8

```
** DIFFICULT TO READ CODE **;
data test ; set orglib.demo ; by inv_no patid ; if patid lt 10 then
do i = 1 to 4 ; subgroup = i ; output ; end ; run ;
proc print data=test ; title 'test data' ; run ;

** EASIER TO READ CODE **;
data test;
set orglib.demo;
by inv_no patid;
if patid lt 10 then do i = 1 to 4;
subgroup = i;
output;
end;
run;
proc print data=test;
title 'test data';
run;
```

While the enhanced SAS editor can help by putting visual lines between steps and procedures, this does not help with statements within a DATA step. In addition, the editor may not always be available to help. For example, you create a program on a UNIX system and use a text editor such as VI or X-Edit to write the code. If this code is printed for review or debugging purposes, the colors will not show up on the printed page. Remember that while the editor is one of many tools available, you should not get in the habit of relying on the editor to debug your program for you. If you write your programs so that the structure of the code itself helps you to understand and debug them, you reduce your validation and maintenance time significantly.

3.5.2.2 Indent Logically

Another structural technique that can help you follow the logic is indention. Your eyes and brain will follow the visual patterns in the code and make it meaningful. Random indention makes code difficult to follow while consistent indention in a logical way makes code easier to read. The code in the next two examples demonstrates how indenting can either help or hinder the ease with which you can follow the logic of program code.

Example 3.9

```
** NOT SO EASY TO READ CODE **;
data test;
        set orglib.demo;
   by inv_no patid;
if patid lt 10 then do i = 1 to 4;
subgroup = i;
   output;
   end;
run;
   proc print data=test;
title 'test data';
        run;
```

Example 3.10

```
** MUCH EASIER TO READ CODE **;
data test;
   set orglib.demo;
   by inv_no patid;
   if patid lt 10 then
   do i = 1 to 4;
      subgroup = i;
      output;
   end;
run;
proc print data=test;
   title 'test data';
run;
```

3.5.2.3 Use White Space to Improve Readability

Another way to increase the readability of code is to add meaningful breaks through the use of white space. Keeping the code reasonably spread out makes it easier to read and discern major logic shifts. For example, keep one blank line between DATA and PROC steps, but add two or three lines when starting a new logical section of code. Data from two separate data sets may be needed to create a table. Putting a few extra blank lines in the code to separate these two sections helps to identify the different sections later. While this may seem inconsequential in simple programs, it becomes more important as programs become longer and more complex. As with many of these techniques, it is possible to overdo. Code should not be run together with no spacing, nor should there be half a page of white space between sections.

3.5.2.4 Use Case to YOUR Advantage

When you are programming, following conventions for using the case of characters makes the program easier to read. While most programmers' initial reaction to this convention is negative ("I don't have time to worry about this stuff!"), if the conventions are kept simple, there is no real reason for objection. For example, all code is typed in lower-case while all comments and procedure titles are typed in uppercase. This convention is easy to follow and immediately allows the programmer to see the difference between real code and extras. While the advanced editor helps to make code easy to read through the use of color, programmers shouldn't get in the habit of relying on the editor to make code readable. Consider the following examples:

Example 3.11

```
** CODE WITHOUT LOGICAL CASE USAGE **;
data TEST;
   set orglib.Demo;
   by INV_NO PATID;
   ** Output one record per subgroup
      for each subject;
   If patid LT 10 then
   DO i = 1 to 4;
      Subgroup = i;
      Output;
   END;
run;
Proc Print data=TEST;
   title 'test data';
RUN;
```

Example 3.12

```
** CODE WITH CASE CONVENTIONS **;
data test;
    set orglib.demo;
    by inv_no patid;
    ** OUTPUT ONE RECORD PER SUBGROUP FOR EACH SUBJECT **;
    if patid lt 10 then
    do i = 1 to 4;
        subgroup = i;
        output;
    end;
run;
proc print data=test;
    title 'TEST DATA';
run;
```

3.5.2.5 Finish What You Start

Place the RUN or QUIT statement where it belongs to visually end each DATA or PROC step. This is the punctuation that ends the sentence or completes the current thought before moving on to the next concept. Even though SAS may not need that statement, it helps the human brain reading the code to process what it's looking at more quickly and easily. Rather than needing to decide if the DATA step has finished, the RUN statement easily confirms it and lets the reader know that both the statement and the concept are finished. In addition, the RUN statement affects where notes appear in the log. By putting the RUN statements at the end of a DATA or PROC step, the notes appear immediately after the RUN statement rather than after the next statement. The log is much easier to read when you are trying to follow observations through program execution or trying to determine where errors are occurring.

3.5.3 One Program, One Purpose

There are four main types of programs used within the statistical programming function for clinical trials—data sets, tables, figures, and data listings. Rather than writing one program per topic, it is much more efficient to write one program per type. For example, in a typical clinical trial, a programmer creates a medical history data set, a summary table, and a data listing. Rather than writing one large medical history program that creates all three of these, it is better to write one program to create the data set, a separate program to create the table, and yet another program to create the data listing.

Keeping the programs compartmental by type makes sense for a number of reasons. First, the data set needs to be created and validated before the table and listing can be created. If a single program contains all three pieces, the data set cannot be validated until the table and listing are finished. Second, if the data set is completed and validated, separate programmers can then simultaneously work on the table and listing. Third, each individual program can be modified (and validated) without the need to revalidate all three pieces of a single program. Finally, programs are much easier to handle when they are separate. If meaningful program naming conventions are followed, it's simple to find the exact program that contains the code needed. It's much simpler to find an appropriately named medical history table (for example, TMH.SAS) than it is to sift through hundreds of lines of code in a single program.

This does not necessarily mean one program per output. While there are few exceptions to the one program, one data set rule, often one program can be used to write multiple tables or multiple listings. A typical example of one program, several listings occurs with adverse events. Often one listing will list serious adverse events, another will list adverse events leading to discontinuation, and yet a third will list adverse events considered related to study medication. Each of these listings has the exact same format; the only difference is the subset of records that is reported. This scenario is the perfect example of where a macro can be placed around the code to pass the subset of records needed so the single program can create all three listings. Notice that the program, while creating three separate output items, creates three very similar outputs from the same source data set. The three listings created are all the same type (listings), deal with the same topic (adverse events), and look very similar.

3.5.4 Comments, Comments, Comments

We've already discussed commenting in programs as a key means to document what the program does and why. Part of maintenance is being able to go back into code and find what is needed to fix, review, or modify quickly and easily. Adding section breaks with comments in the code allows you to do this efficiently. These section breaks describe what each section of code does and can also play a role in making code easy to read visually. To break conceptual sections of code, use comments surrounded by dashes ("--"). For example, "*----- DETERMINE CHANGE FROM BASELINE -----------------*" explains what the next section of code does, but the dashes also provide an easy visual break. While this may not seem important in small programs, these obvious visual breaks are very helpful for larger and more complex programs.

3.5.5 Use Macros Judiciously

The macro is a wonderful tool in SAS, provided it is used judiciously. While macros enable you to make your code more efficient in many ways, they can also make your code more difficult to debug and maintain. For these reasons, always weigh the benefits and the costs of using macros to ensure it is appropriate to use for any given situation. Throughout this book, we discuss various ways that macros can be used to your advantage—and places better suited to using a simpler approach.

3.6 Make Data Maintainable

When programming, it's important that the data as well as the program itself is easy to reference and use. The code that generated the data set won't always be handy as reference when you need to use the data. Thus, it is important to build as much usable information as possible into the data itself. With the increasing adoption of CDISC standards, guidance on how to make data maintainable is more readily available and the prevalence of undocumented data is declining.

3.6.1 Order Your Data

There are two simple ways to bring order to data: the order of the variables and the order of the records. Variables should be stored in the data set in a logical viewing order. In the process of creating variables, the order that they appear in the program data vector is of little concern. As a result, similar or related variables may end up on opposite ends of the data set. For example, the treatment code variable may be the first variable shown in a simple PROC PRINT while the treatment description variable ends up as the eighth variable. This makes looking at the data either with a simple PROC PRINT or through the SAS Viewer difficult.

In addition, the records in a data set should be sorted by the variables that create a unique record. For example, one data set may include the subject ID while another may include subject ID, visit, and test. If data is sorted logically when it is stored, anyone running a PROC CONTENTS statement can easily tell what is needed to find a specific record. Both of these ordering goals can be achieved through a single PROC SQL statement. Using the SELECT statement reorders variables without risk of changing the content of the data itself. The ORDER BY statement sorts the data in the same procedure. To make sure that no key variables are forgotten, using a PROC COMPARE statement of the data set before versus the data set after executing PROC SQL provides the necessary information. Consider the following example:

Example 3.13

```
libname orglib "C:\Book\TestData\Original";
libname sublib "C:\Book\TestData\Submission";
options nodate nocenter noreplace ls=68;

**-----------------------------------------------------------**;
**   GET VARIABLES FROM DEMO DATA                            **;
**-----------------------------------------------------------**;

proc contents data=orglib.demo;
   title 'DEMO DATA FOR PROC CONTENTS EXAMPLE';
run;

data demo;
   length race $25;
   set orglib.demo (drop=barcode pageno proto datestmp e_stat seq);

   length siteid $3 subjid $5 sitesubj $10;

   **   ASSIGN STANDARD CDISC VARIABLES   **;
   studyid = "XYZ4-SAMP-001";
   domain  = 'DM';
   country = 'USA';

   **   GET SITE ID   **;
   siteid = put(inv_no, z2.);

   **   GET SUBJECT ID   **;
   subjid = put(patid, z3.);

   **   GET REPORTED VERSION OF SUBJECT ID   **;
   sitesubj = compress(siteid) || compress(subjid);

   **   GET UNIQUE SUBJECT ID   **;
   usubjid = trim(left(studyid)) || '-' ||
             trim(left(siteid))  || '-' ||
             trim(left(subjid));

   ** CREATE CHARACTER SEX **;
        if sexcd eq 1 then sex = 'M';
   else if sexcd eq 2 then sex = 'F';

   **   COMBINE RACE AND OTHER SPECIFY   **;
   if racecd eq 6 then race = trim(left(raceoth));
                  else race = put(racecd,racecd.);

run;
```

```
proc sort data=demo;
   by sitesubj;
run;

proc print data=demo (obs=5);
   title '5 OBS FROM DEMO WITH CDISC ID VARS ADDED';
run;
```

The first DATA step shown in Example 3.13 creates several new variables based on CDISC guidelines. The resulting output looks like Output 3.2:

Output 3.2

```
5 OBS FROM DEMO WITH CDISC ID VARS ADDED

Obs race              PATID INV_NO SCREENNO SUBJINIT VISIT      BIRTHDT

  8 Hispanic              8    1     1009     RAD     Day -8 10/07/1969
 29 Hispanic             29    1     1038     JRL     Day -8 04/22/1969
125 Hispanic            101    2     2903     AJW     Day -8 12/11/1973
151 CAUCASIAN/ASIAN     175    2     2033     C-D     Day -8 12/28/1976
169 MULTI RACIAL        205    2     2062     SLH     Day -8 04/21/1968


Obs SEXCD    RACECD        RACEOTH      siteid   subjid   sitesubj

  8 2          4                          01      008      01008
 29 2          4                          01      029      01029
125 2          4                          02      101      02101
151 1          6       CAUCASIAN/ASIAN    02      175      02175
169 2          6       MULTI RACIAL       02      205      02205

Obs    studyid     domain   country        usubjid          sex

  8 XYZ4-SAMP-001    DM       USA     XYZ4-SAMP-001-01-008    F
 29 XYZ4-SAMP-001    DM       USA     XYZ4-SAMP-001-01-029    F
125 XYZ4-SAMP-001    DM       USA     XYZ4-SAMP-001-02-101    F
151 XYZ4-SAMP-001    DM       USA     XYZ4-SAMP-001-02-175    M
169 XYZ4-SAMP-001    DM       USA     XYZ4-SAMP-001-02-205    F
```

Notice how the new ID variables are at the end of the presentation—not the ideal. The next piece of code accomplishes several key tasks in one neat step; it reorders the variables into a more logical viewing order, drops unnecessary variables, and sorts the final data set. Immediately following the PROC SQL statement, there is a PROC COMPARE statement to help verify that the content of the final data set is what is expected. The main purpose of this comparison is to show any variables that were missed (either intentionally or by mistake) in the SELECT statement. Note that the LISTALL option must be included in the PROC COMPARE statement in order to get the list of missing variables.

Example 3.14

```
**---------------------------------------------------------------**;
**   OUTPUT SORTED DATA SET                                      **;
**---------------------------------------------------------------**;
options replace;

proc sql;
   create table sublib.dm_ex1 (label='Demographics') as
   select domain, studyid, country, usubjid, siteid, subjid,
          sitesubj, subjinit, visit, sex, race, birthdt
   from demo
   order by sitesubj;
quit;

proc compare base=sublib.dm_ex1 compare=demo listall;
   id sitesubj;
   title "COMPARE OF REORDERED DATA SET";
run;

proc print data=sublib.dm_ex1 (obs=10);
   title "10 OBS FROM OUTGOING DEMO DATA";
run;
```

The resulting output is as follows:

Output 3.3

```
COMPARE OF REORDERED DATA SET

The COMPARE Procedure
Comparison of SUBLIB.DM_EX1 with WORK.DEMO
(Method=EXACT)

Data Set Summary

Dataset                 Created          Modified   NVar   NObs

SUBLIB.DM_EX1  23SEP07:09:10:31  23SEP07:09:10:31     12    244
WORK.DEMO      23SEP07:09:10:31  23SEP07:09:10:31     18    244
```

(*continued*)

```
Variables Summary

Number of Variables in Common: 12.
Number of Variables in WORK.DEMO but not in SUBLIB.DM_EX1: 6.
Number of ID Variables: 1.


Listing of Variables in WORK.DEMO but not in SUBLIB.DM_EX1

Variable  Type  Length  Label

PATID     Num       8   Patient\I.D.
INV_NO    Num       8   Investigator\Number
SCREENNO  Num       4   Screening Number
SEXCD     Num       3   Sex
RACECD    Num       3   Race
RACEOTH   Char     30   Race Specify


Observation Summary

Observation       Base  Compare  ID

First Obs            1        1  sitesubj=01001
Last  Obs          244      244  sitesubj=04228

Number of Observations in Common: 244.
Total Number of Observations Read from SUBLIB.DM_EX1: 244.
Total Number of Observations Read from WORK.DEMO: 244.

Number of Observations with Some Compared Variables Unequal: 0.
Number of Observations with All Compared Variables Equal: 244.

NOTE: No unequal values were found. All values compared are exactly
      equal.
```

The COMPARE output shows that six variables that were in the WORK data set are
not included in the final permanent data set. In this particular case, the variables that
have been omitted were not needed in the final data set (each of these six variables was
reformatted to match the data specifications). The procedure also verifies that no data has
changed between the WORK data set and the final data set. Notice now that when the
data is printed, the variables are presented in a logical order that shows the ID variables
first.

Output 3.4

```
10 OBS FROM OUTGOING DEMO DATA

Obs    domain      studyid       country       usubjid           siteid

  1     DM      XYZ4-SAMP-001      USA      XYZ4-SAMP-001-01-001    01
  2     DM      XYZ4-SAMP-001      USA      XYZ4-SAMP-001-01-002    01
  3     DM      XYZ4-SAMP-001      USA      XYZ4-SAMP-001-01-003    01
  4     DM      XYZ4-SAMP-001      USA      XYZ4-SAMP-001-01-004    01
  5     DM      XYZ4-SAMP-001      USA      XYZ4-SAMP-001-01-005    01
  6     DM      XYZ4-SAMP-001      USA      XYZ4-SAMP-001-01-006    01
  7     DM      XYZ4-SAMP-001      USA      XYZ4-SAMP-001-01-007    01
  8     DM      XYZ4-SAMP-001      USA      XYZ4-SAMP-001-01-008    01
  9     DM      XYZ4-SAMP-001      USA      XYZ4-SAMP-001-01-009    01
 10     DM      XYZ4-SAMP-001      USA      XYZ4-SAMP-001-01-010    01


Obs   subjid   sitesubj   SUBJINIT   VISIT    sex    race       BIRTHDT

  1    001      01001       SAK      Day -8    F    Caucasian   11/25/1946
  2    002      01002       CIS      Day -8    F    Caucasian   01/17/1981
  3    003      01003       MRM      Day -8    F    Caucasian   01/16/1979
  4    004      01004       CMH      Day -8    F    Caucasian   11/01/1972
  5    005      01005       SLV      Day -8    F    Caucasian   04/13/1953
  6    006      01006       CAM      Day -8    M    Caucasian   09/26/1960
  7    007      01007       DAT      Day -8    M    Caucasian   10/13/1969
  8    008      01008       RAD      Day -8    F    Hispanic    10/07/1969
  9    009      01009       SWP      Day -8    M    Caucasian   05/18/1958
 10    010      01010       KAS      Day -8    F    Caucasian   07/09/1960
```

3.6.2 Label Everything

Generally it is common for programmers to assign labels to each data set variable. Especially when limited to eight-character variable names, it is particularly important to label variables meaningfully so the next person looking at the data can figure out what PFSAFO means ("Population flag - safety, original algorithm"). Even though SAS now allows long variable names, the FDA does not accept names over eight characters so the industry standard remains at eight.

In addition to variables, it is also important to add a label to the data set itself. While the name of the data set may seem obvious (MedHx is "Medical History"), larger, more complex studies that collect a lot of different types of data often require more creative and cryptic names. In addition, if CDISC data set naming conventions are followed, all data sets will only have two (per SDTM) or four (per ADaM) character names, such as AE and ADAE. Adding the label option when the data set is created permanently attaches a label to the data set that is shown in PROC CONTENTS output. In Example 3.14, the CREATE TABLE statement in PROC SQL included a LABEL statement. PROC CONTENTS shows the result.

Example 3.15

```
proc contents data=sublib.dm_ex1;
   title "FINAL DEMO DATA SET";
run;
```

Output 3.5

```
FINAL DEMO DATA SET                                                 5

The CONTENTS Procedure

Data Set Name         SUBLIB.DM_EX1        Observations         244
Member Type           DATA                 Variables            12
Engine                V9                   Indexes              0
Created               Sunday, September    Observation Length   104
                      23, 2007 09:13:12 AM
Last Modified         Sunday, September    Deleted Observations 0
                      23, 2007 09:13:12 AM
Protection                                 Compressed           NO
Data Set Type                              Sorted               YES
Label                 Demographics
Data Representation   WINDOWS_32
Encoding              wlatin1  Western
                      (Windows)
Etc...
```

3.6.3 Attach Formats Sparingly

As convenient and useful as user-defined formats can be, they are not an ideal tool when dealing with permanent data sets for this industry. When data sets are exported as transport files or other file types, the formats of the data are not retained—they are unique to SAS data sets. In addition, even if SAS transport files are sent to someone using SAS data sets, the format library may not transfer to SAS used on a different platform. You would need to provide a SAS program to generate the format library at that recipient's site. For the FDA, you cannot assume that all reviewers will be using SAS to look at the data—some may use a tool as simple as Excel.

For these reasons, it is best to refrain from permanently attaching user-defined formats to variables. The convention that has developed is to include both the code variable and the decode variable in the data set. For example, if SEX is coded for sorting in reports

(1=Male, 2=Female), then there would be two variables in the data set—SEXCD (values of 1 and 2) and SEX (values of Male and Female). While this might make programmers accustomed to very normalized data unhappy, it is the easiest way to ensure that the data is usable and understandable by all, regardless of file format. It is, however, acceptable (and recommended) to use standard SAS formats such as date and time formats where appropriate. These formats do not have the same platform-related complications that user-defined formats have and do not impact data import or export.

3.6.4 Consistency Is Key

Regardless of whether you are following CDISC guidelines or some internal standard, it is important to maintain variable name and type consistency across data sets within a study and, more importantly, across studies. As you know, it takes many separate clinical trials to collect enough evidence to gain approval from the FDA. These studies often take years to complete and, in the end, the data from some or all of these studies will be combined into one comprehensive database. It is worth the effort up front to ensure that the variables that contain the same information across all studies are consistent. For example, a variable as simple as SEX can have many variations—numeric with values of 1 and 2, character with values of M and F, or character with values of Male and Female. When three studies are combined, each with differing attributes for the same variable SEX, much more work is required—not only in transforming the data into a consistent format but also researching to confirm the decodes of 1 and 2. If you do a little research in the beginning while you are creating the data sets for an individual study, you will save yourself (or someone else) a lot of work later in the programming and validation process.

3.6.5 Good Housekeeping

In the course of programming, temporary variables are created that are needed only to create or check other variables that will be permanent. Make sure you clean up these variables when you are done with them—especially before storing a permanent data set. If the final product of the program is a permanent data set, additional variables other than those required by the specifications will prevent the data set from passing validation. Even in cases where the final product is a summary table, figure, or listing, dummy variables kept during data processing can cause confusion or even problems when trying to debug. For example, temporary variables left in a data set and then used again for another purpose after a merge with another data set may contain a combination of results from both data sets. Consider the following code and output:

Example 3.16

```
** COUNT EACH SEX **;
data temp ;
   set orglib.demog (keep=site patid sex racecd_) end=lastrec;
   retain cnt1 cnt2 ;
   if sex eq 1 then cnt1+1 ;
   else if sex eq 2 then cnt2+1 ;
   if lastrec then
      do ;
         mcnt = cnt1 ;
         fcnt = cnt2 ;
      end ;
run ;

** COUNT EACH RACE **;
data temp ;
   set temp end=lastrec ;
   retain cnt1 cnt2 ;
   oldcnt1=cnt1 ;   ** THESE 2 LINES FOR EXAMPLE ONLY **;
   oldcnt2=cnt2 ;
   if racecd_ eq 1 then cnt1+1 ;
                   else cnt2+1 ;
   if lastrec then
      do ;
         wcnt = cnt1 ;
         ocnt = cnt2 ;
      end ;
run ;
```

Output 3.6

```
COUNT OF RACE MIXED WITH SEX

                        R                     o    o
                        A                     l    l
             P          C                     d    d
      S      A     S    E    c    c    m    f    c    c    w    o
O     I      T     E    C    n    n    c    c    n    n    c    c
b     T      I     E    D    t    t    n    n    t    t    n    n
s     E      D     X    _    1    2    t    t    1    2    t    t

1     1      1     2    1    1    1    .    .    .    1    .    .
2     1      2     1    1    2    1    .    .    1    1    .    .
3     1      3     2    1    2    2    .    .    1    2    .    .
4     1      4     2    1    2    3    .    .    1    3    .    .
```

(continued)

5	1	10	2	1	2	4	.	.	1	4	.	.
6	2	1	1	2	2	5	.	.	2	4	.	.
7	2	2	2	1	3	5	.	.	2	5	.	.
8	2	3	1	1	4	5	.	.	3	5	.	.
9	2	4	1	9	4	6	.	.	4	5	.	.
10	2	5	1	1	6	5	.	.	5	5	.	.
11	**2**	**10**	**1**	**2**	**6**	**6**	**6**	**5**	**6**	**5**	**6**	**6**

In this example, two items (SEX and RACE) are being counted in two different DATA steps for ultimate use in a summary table. The final results for the table would be contained in the last record, but all records are kept in this example to show what is happening within the DATA step. While this code example is meant for simplicity, it is easy to extrapolate to a much more complex coding task. If the temporary variables used to count in the first DATA step had been dropped once the processing was finished, the results from the second data set would have been correct (WCNT would have been 8 and OCNT would have been 3). In addition to making the printed output more difficult to review when trying to debug, in this case the temporary variables left in the data set cause errors in the logic later in the program. Simple DROP statements like the one here can prevent both of these from happening:

```
data temp (drop=cnt1 cnt2);
```

3.6.6 Look—but Don't Touch

One of the cardinal rules of statistical programming is never to hard-code changes to the data. Simply put, hard-coding is changing the value and meaning of a data point through the use of a program outside of a CFR Part 11-compliant data management system. Essentially, this is changing data without the use of an approved audit trail. While it is often easy to tell what constitutes hard-coding, other times it is not so obvious. Consider the following data set:

Output 3.7

```
DEMOG DATA FOR HARDCODE EXAMPLE

                                      R
                                R     A
                                A     C                   H      W      T
                        P       C     E                   E      E      R
                 S      A       E     S                   I      I      T
         O       I      T         D S C     P             G      G      M
         b       T      I         O E D     E             H      H      N
         s       E      D         B X _     C             T      T      T

         1       1      1    25NOV1946  2 1              170.2   60.3   1
         2       1      2    01NOV1972  1 1              170.2   76.2   2
         3       1      3    13OCT1969  2 1              165.1   69.3   1
         4       1      4    18MAY1958  2 1              184.2  114.8   2
         5       1     10    24MAY1999  2 1              182.9   90.3   1
         6       2      1    15MAR1974  1 2              167.6  105.2   1
         7       2      2    04JAN1983  2 1              165.1   64.0   2
         8       2      3    22DEC1963  1 1              167.6   81.6   1
         9       2      4    28DEC1976  1 9  CAUCASIAN/ASIAN 167.6   59.6   2
        10       2      5    04OCT1958  1 1              170.2   77.1   1
        11       2     10    05JUL1969  1 2              158.8   61.0   2
```

Notice in the data above that Site 1, Subject 2 is SEX 1 while all other subjects at that site are SEX 2 and vice-versa with Site 2, Subject 2. Now consider the following code:

Example 3.17

```
proc format;
    value racecd 1 = 'Caucasian'
                 2 = 'Black'
                 3 = 'Asian'
                 9 = 'Other';
run;

data demo;
    set inlib.demog (rename=(sex=sexcd));

    ** SCENARIO 1 **;
         if site eq 1 and patid eq 2 then sexcd = 2;
    else if site eq 2 and patid eq 2 then sexcd = 1;
```

```
** SCENARIO 2 **;
     if site eq 1 then sexcd = 2;
else if site eq 2 then sexcd = 1;

** SCENARIO 3 **;
length sex $6;
     if sexcd eq 1 then sex = 'Male';
else if sexcd eq 2 then sex = 'Female';

** SCENARIO 4 **;
length race $40;
if racecd_ ne 9 then race = put(racecd_,racecd.);
                else race = racespec;

run;
```

Scenario 1 is the most obvious and easy-to-discern example of hard-coding. It is quite obviously changing the meaning of a specific data point. While Scenario 2 may look a little safer, the end result is the same—the fundamental meaning of select data points is being changed. In this case, if only the code were reviewed and not the data, the hard-coding would not be obvious. Both of these scenarios are considered equally unacceptable. Scenarios 3 and 4, while reformatting the existing data, do not change the underlying meaning of it. This type of code is acceptable and often necessary to enable you to store and report the data as required.

Although hard-coding is fundamentally unacceptable, there are cases where it is necessary. Take the example above—assume that the data is from an old study (finished 2 years ago) and there is no way to change the data through a data management system. This data is being combined with other studies and through researching the original CRFs, a data entry error is discovered—the SEX for Site 1, Subject 2 got switched with Site 2, Subject 2. The only way to fix this true error in the data is through hard-coding. In these cases, it is important to document that the data was changed both within the code and externally in an appropriate regulatory document. Provided there is evidence to support the need for the change (and what that change should be) and there is adequate documentation, hard-coding can be performed in exceptional circumstances.

3.7 Conclusion

All of the techniques discussed in this chapter may seem like a lot to remember. It may also appear that some of the information in this chapter is either commonplace or over-kill. Keep in mind that while these concepts are described in simple situations here, as programs become more involved and complex, they are much more critical. Documentation is a necessity, both for ensuring programming output is accurate and for providing evidence that validation was performed based on an SOP or other guideline. Creating code that is easy to read and maintain can facilitate validation, both for the immediate need and for any future requirements. While these techniques may seem to take more time up front, they invariably save time over the course of a trial or set of trials. By helping the validation process move more smoothly, the final output can reach its destination more quickly and—more importantly—more accurately.

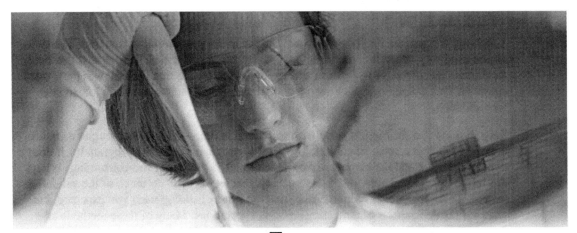

C h a p t e r **4**

General Techniques to Facilitate Validation

4.1 Introduction

Validation is a process that occurs throughout the entire programming function. The techniques used vary depending on the actual activity being performed. Throughout this book, we discuss specific ways to perform tasks and ways to ensure that the task was performed correctly. This chapter offers an overview of some general techniques and philosophies for validation.

Keep in mind that the biggest issue with validation is time—clients want output as quickly as possible, but it must be correct. You need to program so that the program itself does most of the work and the manual review time (which is the most time-consuming) is kept to a minimum. This chapter discusses methods that let the code do much of the validation for you. These techniques help to ensure that the syntax is doing what you expected, but often syntax depends on data meeting certain expectations. Many of these methods address both issues at once—they show that the logic is working and that the data meets the assumptions made by that logic.

4.2 Validation Tools

SAS provides a host of methods to help validate code and data. Most are simple to use; it's just a matter of knowing how to use them to your best advantage. Let's discuss some of the more commonly used tools that are available as well as how to use them efficiently for validation.

4.2.1 Procedures

There are a wide variety of procedures provided within SAS that help do everything from sorting data to generating complex statistical analyses. While most people tend to think of the more complex procedures and how to use them, it is the simple procedures that are most helpful for validation of data and logic.

4.2.1.1 Using PROC PRINT to Display Subsets of Data

PROC PRINT is most helpful when working with small amounts of data. However, it can also be helpful when used selectively with larger data sets. While most programmers first think of PROC CONTENTS for understanding what is in a data set, PROC PRINT gives you a different and equally important view of the data. Often the structure of the data set does not offer a clear picture of what it actually contains. However, simply printing entire data sets is not always helpful either—especially when most data sets are hundreds of observations long and take dozens of pages to print. A key technique to using PROC PRINT in the pharmaceutical industry is printing *select* observations both before and after the data has been manipulated. This output is then used to show that the data was not changed inappropriately. Most often, observations are selected by a subject identifier and that subject's data is printed both before and after it is manipulated. Also, it is customary to select several subjects' data for validation—usually at least one "clean" subject and several that may have issues or "odd" data combinations that will hit different logic areas in the code. With the addition of a little help from SAS macros, this is simple to accomplish.

Using the macro language identifier %LET, create a macro variable that contains all of the values of the subject identifiers. Using PROC PRINT and the WHERE operator, subset the data to print only the subjects in the &VALPATS macro variable.

Example 4.1

```
%let valpats=patid in(1 3 8);

proc print data = orglib.demo (where=(&valpats)) ;
   title 'INCOMING DATA';
run;
data demo2;
   set orglib.demo;
   length sitesubj $7;
   sitesubj = put(inv_no,z3.) || '-' || put(patid, z3.);
run;
proc print data = demo2 (where=(&valpats));
   title 'DATA AFTER MANIPULATION';
run;
```

The results appear in Output 4.1.

Output 4.1

```
INCOMING DATA

Obs      INV_NO      PATID

  1         1          1
  3         1          3
  8         1          8

DATA AFTER MANIPULATION

Obs      INV_NO      PATID      sitesubj

  1         1          1        001-001
  3         1          3        001-003
  8         1          8        001-008
```

The results display only observations where the subject identifier is equal to 1, 3, or 8.

PROC PRINT is also useful when printing *select* records from large data sets. In Example 4.2, the vital signs data set has more than 1,700 records—it's very impractical to print the entire data set. However, records of interest are those with missing data (there are 4 missing values, .A through .Z and .).

Example 4.2

```
proc print data=vitals(where=(sysbp lt .Z));
   var inv_no patid visit sysbp diabp resp pr;
   title "MISSING VITAL SIGNS?!";
run;
```

The results of printing select records from a large data set are shown in Output 4.2.

Output 4.2

```
MISSING VITAL SIGNS?!

  Obs    INV_NO    PATID    VISIT     SYSBP    DIABP    RESP    PR

    4        1        1     Week 2      N        N        N      N
  722        2       79     Week 2      N        N        N      N
  832        2       94     Week 4      N        N        N      N
 1543        4      143     Week 6      N        N        N      N
```

Another way that PROC PRINT is very helpful for data validation is through use of the cell index. A cell index is utilized in programs that produce summary statistics. It details each subject's data that contributed to the summary statistic. In the following example, the program produces a report with summary counts of the number of subjects with a history of abnormalities in each body system. Each subject can be counted only once in each body system. The initial sort removes any possible duplicates and sorts the data appropriately for the cell index. The subsequent PROC PRINT uses both the BY and ID statements with the same variable, which produces a grouped listing. The N option produces a group total. Notice that this technique can produce a significant amount of output and will often need to be subset to a specific subcategory when working with larger data sets.

Example 4.3

```
proc sort data=orglib.medhist (where=(mhstatcd eq 1))
          out=body
          nodupkey;
   by mhbodsys inv_no patid;
run;

proc print data=body n;
   where mhbodsys in('HEMATOLOGIC/ONCOLOGIC' 'HEPATIC/RENAL');
   by mhbodsys;
   id mhbodsys;
   var inv_no patid;
   title "SUBJECTS GOING INTO TOTAL BODY SYSTEM COUNTS";
run;
```

Output 4.3 shows the cell index produced by Example 4.3.

Output 4.3

```
SUBJECTS GOING INTO TOTAL BODY SYSTEM COUNTS

MHBODSYS                    INV_NO    PATID

HEMATOLOGIC/ONCOLOGIC          1          5
                               1         11
                               1         18
                               1         20
                               1         21
                               1         38
                               1        220
                               2         45
                               2         99
                               2        103
                               2        167
                               2        170
                               2        174
                               2        176
                               2        242
                               3        132
                               3        135
                               3        216
                               3        236
                               4        146
                               4        158


N = 21

HEPATIC/RENAL                  1         21
                               1         26
                               1         31
                               1        233
                               2         58
                               2         70
                               2         75
                               2         78
                               2         87
                               2         89
                               2        104
                               2        105
                               2        164
                               2        172
                               2        244
                               4        148
                               4        154
                               4        160

N = 18
```

The next section of code produces the summary counts that will appear in the final report. Notice that PROC FREQ produces an output data set only. Displaying this data set with PROC PRINT shows exactly what the underlying data looks like.

Example 4.4

```
proc freq data=body noprint;
   table mhbodsys / missing out=bsyscnt (drop=percent);
run;

proc print data=bsyscnt;
   title "COUNTS OF BODY SYSTEM";
run;
```

Output 4.4 shows summary counts created by Example 4.4.

Output 4.4

```
COUNTS OF BODY SYSTEM

Obs     MHBODSYS                          COUNT

  1     ALLERGIC DISORDERS                  108
  2     CARDIOVASCULAR                       30
  3     CNS                                 103
  4     DERMATOLOGIC                         42
  5     GASTROINTESTINAL                     79
  6     GENITOURINARY/GYNECOLOGICAL         100
  7     HEENT                               136
  8     HEMATOLOGIC/ONCOLOGIC                21
  9     HEPATIC/RENAL                        18
 10     METABOLIC/ENDOCRINE                  24
 11     OTHER                               114
 12     PULMONARY                            22
```

Notice that the Hematologic/Oncologic body system indicates that there are 21 subjects with an abnormality in this group. If another individual checking counts finds only 20 subjects, you would each need to know which subjects went into the counts to determine where the discrepancy is. The cell index produced by PROC PRINT prior to creating the summary statistic provides a fast and simple way to perform this check.

4.2.1.2 Using PROC FREQ for Validation

PROC FREQ is most commonly used in clinical data validation when categorical data needs to be recoded. Often, categorical data is collected as numeric codes when specifications require text to be stored in the data set. Data from two variables may be combined into one, such as the example of a coded RACE variable and a separate "other, specify" variable. It may simply be a matter of creating a character version of a variable that was originally collected as a numeric code, as in the case of the SEX variable. In either case, code needs to prove that the meaning of the variables being transformed has not changed. The code must show that in every case where SEXCD was "1", SEX is now "Male", and in every case where SEXCD was "2", SEX is now "Female". When you are performing cross-variable checks, it is most helpful to view PROC FREQ output in list format as Example 4.5 demonstrates.

Example 4.5

```
data demo;
   set orglib.demo;
        if sexcd eq 1 then sex = "Male";
   else if sexcd eq 2 then sex = "Female";
   if racecd ne 6 then race = put(racecd, racecd.);
   else race = "Other";
run;

proc freq data=demo;
   tables racecd*race sexcd*sex / list missing nopercent nocum;
   title 'CHECK RECODES';
run;
```

Output 4.5 displays the PROC FREQ output for checking variable recoding.

Output 4.5

```
CHECK RECODES

The FREQ Procedure

RACECD    race          Frequency
-------------------------------
     1    Caucasian          215
     2    Black               19
     3    Asian                4
     4    Hispanic             3
     6    Other                3
```

(continued)

```
SEXCD    sex      Frequency
--------------------------
   1    Male           78
   2    Fema          166
```

In this output, it is easy to spot the error in reformatting the SEXCD variable—the
LENGTH statement was omitted from the code in Example 4.5; therefore, the length
of SEX defaulted to the length of the first value, 4. This is an easy mistake to make and
PROC FREQ can help spot this type of mistake quickly.

PROC FREQ can also be used to check continuous data. In order for this to be practical, you need to use PROC FORMAT. In most cases, PROC FREQ is used with PROC
FORMAT to check continuous variables for values that are out of range, including dates.
This is useful to verify that data values are reasonable. It can catch cases where the unit of
measure in which the data was supposed to be collected was not how the data was actually collected. It is also helpful for catching any data entry errors that may have slipped
through the database cleaning process.

Example 4.6

```
proc format;
   value chknums   . - .Z = 'MISSING'
                 low - <0 = 'negative'
                        0 = 'ZERO'
                 0<-high = 'positive'
                    other = 'other???'
                    ;
   value chkbyten . - .Z = 'MISSING'
                 low -<0 = 'negative'
                        0 = 'ZERO'
                  0<-10 = '>0 - 10'
                 10<-20 = '>10 - 20'
                 20<-30 = '>20 - 30'
                 30<-40 = ,>30 - 40'
                 40<-50 = ,>40 - 50'
                        etc.
                    other = 'over 200?!'
                    ;
   value chkdate   . - .Z      = '<<MISSING>>'
                 LOW - -21915 = 'Pre-1900?!'
               -21914- -18263 = '1900s'
               -18262- -14611 = '1910s'
               -14610- -10958 = '1920s'
               -10957-  -7306 = '1930s'
                -7305 -  -3653 = '1940s'
                -3652 -    -1 = '1950s'
```

```
                      0 -    3652 = '1960s'
               3653 -    7304 = '1970s'
               7305 -   10957 = '1980s'
              10958 -   14609 = '1990s'
              14610 -   16802 = '2000 - 2005'
              16803 -   17030 = '2006'
              17031 -   %sysfunc(today()) = '2007'
              %sysfunc(today()) - HIGH = 'FUTURE?!'
                  ;
    run;

    proc freq data=orglib.vitals;
       format sysbp diabp chkbyten.;
       table sysbp / missing list nopercent;
       title "CHECK SYSTOLIC BP ON ORIGINAL VITALS DATA";
    run;

    proc freq data=orglib.visit;
       format actdt chkdate.;
       table actdt / missing list nopercent;
       title "CHECK VISIT DATES";
    run;
```

The PROC FREQ results on continuous variables using PROC FORMAT is shown in Output 4.6.

Output 4.6

```
CHECK SYSTOLIC BP ON ORIGINAL VITALS DATA


The FREQ Procedure

        Sitting Systolic BP

                          Cumulative
      SYSBP    Frequency   Frequency
-------------------------------------
MISSING            4           4
>70 - 80           4           8
>80 - 90          25          33
>90 - 100        219         252
>100 - 110       532         784
>110 - 120       496        1280
>120 - 130       290        1570
```

(continued)

```
>130 - 140          108          1678
>140 - 150           38          1716
>150 - 160            9          1725
>170 - 180            1          1726
over 200              1          1727


CHECK VISIT DATES


The FREQ Procedure


                Visit Date


                              Cumulative
      ACTDT     Frequency      Frequency
-------------------------------------------
1900s               1                  1
2000 - 2005      1728               1729
FUTURE?!            1               1730
```

It is easy to find the outlying values that may need to be reviewed in more detail. Once these values are discovered, the appropriate observations can be printed for closer inspection.

4.2.2 SAS Options and Language Elements

In addition to procedures, SAS has a number of options and DATA step elements that can help programmers check data. One of the most common ways to check or manipulate data is to merge two data sets together. Using the SAS option MSGLEVEL=I and the IN= option on data sets being merged are two key elements that help to ensure data merges correctly. However, in order for these options to be effective, you need to check the program log—and not just for warning or error messages. In the example below, note that the names of the IN= variables start with "in" to differentiate these temporary variables from data set variables. The assumption when merging these two data sets is that there is a one-to-one match. Review of the observation counts in the resulting log shows that this was not the case.

The code contains no syntax errors, but where did the observations go?

Output 4.7

```
212          data vitals;
213             merge vitals(in=invl)
214                   visit (in=invt)
215                   ;
216             by inv_no patid visit;
217             if invl and invt then output vitals;
218          run;

NOTE: There were 1727 observations read from the data set WORK.VITALS.
NOTE: There were 1726 observations read from the data set WORK.VISIT.
NOTE: The data set WORK.VITALS has 1723 observations and 19 variables.
NOTE: DATA statement used (Total process time):
      real time            0.01 seconds
      cpu time             0.01 seconds
```

The MSGLEVEL system option gives additional information in the log when merging data sets. When this option is set to "I", it produces information lines in the log that inform the programmer when variables occur in both data sets being merged. In SAS 6, all variables are listed; however, after SAS 8, only variables not included in the BY statement are listed. The next example shows another technique for using the IN= option. Using these temporary variables, you can direct unexpected merge results to separate data sets so that problem records are identified and any issues can be resolved.

Example 4.7

```
options msglevel=I;
data vitals checkme;
   merge vitals(in=invl)
         visit (in=invt);
   by inv_no patid visit;
   if invl and invt then output vitals;
                    else output checkme;
run;
```

When these data sets are merged, SAS outputs to the log any variables that exist in both data sets and that are being overwritten. In this example, variables INV_NO, PATID, VISIT, BARCODE, and SEQ are in both data sets. Because the BY statement includes INV_NO, PATID, and VISIT, SAS expects them to be in both. However, the variables BARCODE and SEQ are not in the BY statement, so SAS informs you that values are going to be overwritten.

Log results with MSGLEVEL=I are shown in Output 4.8.

Output 4.8

```
237        data vitals checkme;
238           merge vitals(in=invl)
239                 visit (in=invt);
240           by inv_no patid visit;
241           if invl and invt then output vitals;
242                          else output checkme;
243        run;

INFO: The variable BARCODE on data set WORK.VITALS will be overwritten
      by data set WORK.VISIT.
INFO: The variable SEQ on data set WORK.VITALS will be overwritten
      by data set WORK.VISIT.
NOTE: There were 1727 observations read from the data set WORK.VITALS.
NOTE: There were 1730 observations read from the data set WORK.VISIT.
NOTE: The data set WORK.VITALS has 1727 observations and 16 variables.
NOTE: The data set WORK.CHECKME has 3 observations and 16 variables.
NOTE: DATA statement used (Total process time):
      real time          0.01 seconds
      cpu time           0.01 seconds
```

The log is one of the most useful debugging tools provided by SAS. With the implementation of SAS 8, the log has become even more helpful. With enhanced system options and more output from which to choose, it is really only a matter of understanding what to analyze.

4.2.2.1 Merging Data to Itself

A SAS tip that many programmers don't think about is to merge data to itself. Merging data to itself is very efficient because you don't need to create extra data sets and all of the features of a DATA step are available to check that the merge happened as expected. Consider the following scenario: There is an analytic need to count the number of people in each treatment group (in this example, there are two groups). Begin by counting the number of people in each treatment group using the SAFETY variable (the population flag denoting the safety population). Counting the subject number produces a record for each subject. Counting the SAFETY variable produces the total number in each treatment group.

Example 4.8

```
proc freq data=demo;
   table trtcd*safety / out=totsafe (drop=percent) noprint;
run;
```

```
proc print data=totsafe;
    title 'SAFETY POPULATION COUNTS FROM PROC FREQ';
run;
```

The output from the code in this example is displayed below. Notice that there are no patients in the second treatment group with a SAFETY value of "N".

Output 4.9

```
SAFETY POPULATION COUNTS FROM PROC FREQ

Obs     trtcd     safety     COUNT

 1        1          N          3
 2        1          Y         135
 3        2          Y         106
```

For the output we need to create, TRTCD needs to be a column while SAFETY remains a row. In most cases, you could use PROC TRANSPOSE, which would result in Output 4.10.

Example 4.9

```
proc transpose data=totsafe out=transtot prefix=trt;
    by safety;
    id trtcd;
    var count;
run;

proc print data=transtot;
    title "TRANSPOSED TOTSAFE FROM PROC TRANSPOSE";
run;
```

Output 4.10

```
TRANSPOSED TOTSAFE FROM PROC TRANSPOSE

Obs     safety     _NAME_          _LABEL_          trt_1     trt_2

 1        N         COUNT      Frequency Count        3         .
 2        Y         COUNT      Frequency Count       135       106
```

While this result is correct, notice the missing value under TRT_2. This data needs to be processed through another DATA step before being reported because the count in this cell is not really missing. It is zero. In addition, other than providing warnings when data cannot be processed correctly, PROC TRANSPOSE does not have any means to check the resulting output. Consider the alternative in Example 4.10.

Example 4.10

```
data mrgtot (drop = trtcd) check;
   merge totsafe (where=(trtcd = 1) rename=(count = trt_1))
         totsafe (where=(trtcd = 2) rename=(count = trt_2));
   by safety;
   if trt_1 eq . and safety eq 'N' then trt_1 = 0;
   if trt_2 eq . and safety eq 'N' then trt_2 = 0;
   if (trt_1 eq . or trt_2 eq .) and safety eq 'Y' then output
check;
   else output mrgtot;
run;

proc print data=check;
   title 'TREATEMENT GROUP WITH NO SAFETY EVAL PATIENTS - ISSUE?';
run;

proc print data=mrgtot;
   title 'TRANSPOSED TOTSAFE FROM DATA STEP MERGE';
run;
```

In this DATA statement, the BY variable (TRTCD) is dropped. This variable is no longer needed because we now have the data in a horizontal fashion, with treatment groups as variables. The TRTCD variable is not needed. In addition, there is now added logic to check for unexpected missing values, as well as code to change expected missing values to zero. In this example, no records fell into the CHECK data set, but it is easy to see how this method of transposing data can be used to make the code do the bulk of the work during the validation process.

As a result, the data set MRGTOT appears as follows:

Output 4.11

```
TRANSPOSED TOTSAFE FROM DATA STEP MERGE

Obs     safety     trt_1      trt_2

1         N           3          0
2         Y         135        106
```

4.2.3 Using Macros Effectively

Macros are a powerful tool within SAS that can be a great asset for validation. Like all powerful tools, macros need to be used appropriately. Macros can also create validation nightmares when used in excess. The general rule for truly efficient programming is to use macros only when they add significantly to the process. Writing a simple, straight-forward piece of code and then encapsulating it within a %MACRO–%MEND structure is not in itself an appropriate use of this powerful SAS feature. However, a simple piece of code that is used repeatedly throughout many programs makes it more appropriate for macro usage.

Throughout the course of a program, you print records that could contain data issues. The code is very simple, as follows:

Example 4.11

```
proc print data = check;
   Title "CHECK: POTENTIAL DATA ISSUE";
run;
```

Putting code like this into a macro would normally be considered macro overkill; how-ever, by putting this common piece of code into a macro, you can add some nice features that make it worth the added effort. While this code does print data issues and the log will show if any observations were selected, often it is easier to look for specific warn-ing messages in the log. Using the macro language enhances this simple code example as follows:

Example 4.12

```
/*****************************************************************
    MACRO: MCHECK
    PURPOSE: PRINT CHECKING DATA SET AND PUT WARNING IN LOG
    PARAMETERS:  INSET = NAME OF DATA SET TO PRINT
                 WHY   = TITLE FOR PRINT OUTPUT
*****************************************************************/
%macro mcheck(inset=check,why=);

   /* IF CHECK DATASET HAS OBS THEN PRINT AND WARN IN LOG */
   data _null_;
      if 0 then set &inset nobs=numobs;
      call symput("CCCC", left(put(numobs,5.)));
      stop;
   run;

   %if &cccc ne 0 %then
      %do;
```

```
        proc print data=&inset;
            title "WHOOPS: &why";
        run;
        title;
        %put WARNING: &why;
    %end;

%mend mcheck;
```

The macro code in Example 4.12 has the added feature of including a warning message in the log and, as a result, makes it easier to spot issues during the validation process. Again, this would not necessarily be worth the effort to incorporate into a macro, but the fact that this code is used frequently throughout many programs makes it worthwhile. When you are deciding whether to introduce the complication of macros, it is always important to consider the cost-benefit ratio. Will you gain significant time or efficiency for the added complication? If the answer is yes, macros are a powerful tool that will add to the programming process.

If macros are appropriate for a given task, there are several SAS options that can make validating and debugging macro code much easier. These options help show how code moves through the macro processor and can offer insight into why an error or unintended result occurred. These options are discussed in the next few pages.

4.2.3.1 Using MPRINT to Validate Macros

Perhaps one of the most useful tools for validating and debugging macros is the MPRINT option. This option shows the code that results after the macro processor is finished and allows notes in the log to follow the DATA or PROC step that they are associated with. Consider the following code:

Example 4.13

```
%macro dostuff(invar=,cutoff=);
    data d&invar dropped;
        set vitals;
        by inv_no patid;
        retain &invar.flag;
        if first.patid then &invar.flag = .;
            if &invar lt &cutoff and &invar.flag lt 2 then &invar.flag=1;
        else if &invar ge &cutoff                        then &invar.flag=2;
        if not last.patid then output dropped;
                      else output d&invar;
    run;
```

```
proc print data=d&invar (obs=10);
    var inv_no patid visit &invar &invar.flag;
    title "PTS WITH &INVAR SEVERITY FLAG CUTOFF OF &CUTOFF (10 OBS)";
run;
proc print data=dropped;
    var inv_no patid visit &invar &invar.flag;
    title "DUPLICATES DROPPED - CHECK SEVERITY FLAG FOR &INVAR";
run;
%mend;
%dostuff(invar=pr,cutoff=100)
```

The log that results from running this code without the MPRINT option is shown in
Output 4.12.

Output 4.12

```
477          %macro dostuff(invar=,cutoff=);
478             data d&invar dropped;
479                set vitals;
480                by inv_no patid;
481                retain &invar.flag;
482                if first.patid then &invar.flag = .;
483                     if &invar lt &cutoff and &invar.flag lt 2 then
483      !   &invar.flag = 1;
484                else if &invar ge &cutoff                    then
484      !   &invar.flag = 2;
485                if not last.patid then output dropped;
486                                else output d&invar;
487             run ;
488             proc print data=d&invar (obs=10);
489                var inv_no patid visit &invar &invar.flag;
490                title "PATIENTS WITH &INVAR OVER SEVERITY FLAG
490      ! CUTOFF OF &CUTOFF (10 OBS)";
491             run;
492             proc print data=dropped;
493                var inv_no patid visit &invar &invar.flag;
494                title "DUPLICATES DROPPED - CHECK SEVERITY FLAG FOR
494      !   &INVAR";
495             run;
496          %mend;
497
498          %dostuff(invar=pr,cutoff=100)
```

(continued)

```
NOTE: There were 1727 observations read from the data set WORK.
      VITALS.
NOTE: The data set WORK.DPR has 244 observations and 19 variables.
NOTE: The data set WORK.DROPPED has 1483 observations and 19
      variables.
NOTE: DATA statement used (Total process time):
      real time              0.07 seconds
      cpu time               0.01 seconds




NOTE: There were 10 observations read from the data set WORK.DPR.
NOTE: The PROCEDURE PRINT printed page 27.
NOTE: PROCEDURE PRINT used (Total process time):
      real time              0.01 seconds
      cpu time               0.01 seconds



NOTE: There were 1483 observations read from the data set WORK.
      DROPPED.
NOTE: The PROCEDURE PRINT printed pages 28-57.
NOTE: PROCEDURE PRINT used (Total process time):
      real time              0.01 seconds
      cpu time               0.01 seconds
```

Notice that there are notes in the log describing the results of the DATA step and prints, but these notes are totally unconnected to the code itself. In addition, there is no way to know how each of the macro variables embedded in the code resolved. With the MPRINT option, the log is much more readable.

Output 4.13

```
500         options mprint;
501
502         %dostuff(invar=pr,cutoff=100)
MPRINT(DOSTUFF):   data dpr dropped;
MPRINT(DOSTUFF):   set vitals;
MPRINT(DOSTUFF):   by inv_no patid;
MPRINT(DOSTUFF):   retain prflag;
MPRINT(DOSTUFF):   if first.patid then prflag = .;
MPRINT(DOSTUFF):   if pr lt 100 and prflag lt 2 then prflag = 1;
MPRINT(DOSTUFF):   else if pr ge 100 then prflag = 2;
MPRINT(DOSTUFF):   if not last.patid then output dropped;
MPRINT(DOSTUFF):   else output dpr;
MPRINT(DOSTUFF):   run;
```

(*continued*)

```
NOTE: There were 1727 observations read from the data set WORK.
      VITALS.
NOTE: The data set WORK.DPR has 244 observations and 19 variables.
NOTE: The data set WORK.DROPPED has 1483 observations and 19
      variables.
NOTE: DATA statement used (Total process time):
      real time            0.09 seconds
      cpu time             0.00 seconds


MPRINT(DOSTUFF):    proc print data=dpr (obs=10);
MPRINT(DOSTUFF):    var inv_no patid visit pr prflag;
MPRINT(DOSTUFF):    title "PTS WITH pr SEVERITY FLAG CUTOFF OF 100
                    (10 OBS)";
MPRINT(DOSTUFF):    run;

NOTE: There were 10 observations read from the data set WORK.DPR.
NOTE: The PROCEDURE PRINT printed page 58.
NOTE: PROCEDURE PRINT used (Total process time):
      real time            0.01 seconds
      cpu time             0.01 seconds


MPRINT(DOSTUFF):    proc print data=dropped;
MPRINT(DOSTUFF):    var inv_no patid visit pr prflag;
MPRINT(DOSTUFF):    title "DUPLICATES DROPPED - CHECK SEVERITY FLAG
                    FOR pr";
MPRINT(DOSTUFF):    run;

NOTE: There were 1483 observations read from the data set WORK.
      DROPPED.
NOTE: The PROCEDURE PRINT printed pages 59-88.
NOTE: PROCEDURE PRINT used (Total process time):
      real time            0.00 seconds
      cpu time             0.00 seconds
```

While the need to see exactly how the macro variables resolve might not seem important when the code is working correctly, it is invaluable in cases where it is not.

4.2.3.2 Using SYMBOLGEN

Another system option that is useful for debugging macro code is SYMBOLGEN. This option is particularly helpful when the value of a macro variable determines whether code is generated for the SAS compiler. In these instances, MPRINT is not helpful because it does not generate code and, as a result, nothing appears in the log. Consider the following example where, depending on the value of &VALID (a macro variable that is not defined within the macro programmed here), whole sections of code might not be executed. In this example, &VALID is set to 0 and, therefore, the PRINT procedures do not execute. The SYMBOLGEN option allows the highlighted row to be printed in the log, which explains why the code did not execute. In more complex code, this helps determine if macro code is being executed properly.

Example 4.14

```
%macro dostuff(invar=,cutoff=);
   data d&invar dropped;
      set vitals;
      by inv_no patid;
      retain &invar.flag;
      if first.patid then &invar.flag = .;
           if &invar lt &cutoff and &invar.flag lt 2 then &invar.flag=1;
      else if &invar ge &cutoff                       then &invar.flag=2;
      if not last.patid then output dropped;
                      else output d&invar;
   run;
   %if &valid=1 %then
   %do;
      proc print data=d&invar (obs=10);
         var inv_no patid visit &invar &invar.flag;
         title "PTS W/&INVAR SEVERITY FLAG CUTOFF=&CUTOFF (10 OBS)";
      run;
      proc print data=dropped;
         var inv_no patid visit &invar &invar.flag;
         title "DUPLICATES DROPPED - CHECK SEVERITY FLAG FOR &INVAR";
      run;
   %end;
%mend;

options symbolgen;
%dostuff(invar=pr,cutoff=100)
```

Output 4.14

```
533        %dostuff(invar=pr,cutoff=100)
SYMBOLGEN:  Macro variable INVAR resolves to pr
MPRINT(DOSTUFF):   data dpr dropped;
MPRINT(DOSTUFF):   set vitals;
MPRINT(DOSTUFF):   by inv_no patid;
SYMBOLGEN:  Macro variable INVAR resolves to pr
MPRINT(DOSTUFF):   retain prflag;
SYMBOLGEN:  Macro variable INVAR resolves to pr
MPRINT(DOSTUFF):   if first.patid then prflag = .;
SYMBOLGEN:  Macro variable INVAR resolves to pr
SYMBOLGEN:  Macro variable CUTOFF resolves to 100
SYMBOLGEN:  Macro variable INVAR resolves to pr
SYMBOLGEN:  Macro variable INVAR resolves to pr
MPRINT(DOSTUFF):   if pr lt 100 and prflag lt 2 then prflag = 1;
SYMBOLGEN:  Macro variable INVAR resolves to pr
SYMBOLGEN:  Macro variable CUTOFF resolves to 100
SYMBOLGEN:  Macro variable INVAR resolves to pr
MPRINT(DOSTUFF):   else if pr ge 100 then prflag = 2;
MPRINT(DOSTUFF):   if not last.patid then output dropped;
SYMBOLGEN:  Macro variable INVAR resolves to pr
MPRINT(DOSTUFF):   else output dpr;
MPRINT(DOSTUFF):   run;
NOTE: There were 1727 observations read from the data set
      WORK.VITALS.
NOTE: The data set WORK.DPR has 244 observations and 19 variables.
NOTE: The data set WORK.DROPPED has 1483 observations and 19
      variables.
NOTE: DATA statement used (Total process time):
      real time            0.01 seconds
      cpu time             0.01 seconds

SYMBOLGEN:  Macro variable VALID resolves to 0
```

Because the SYMBOLGEN option generates a large number of additional lines in the log, it is not often left on for the entire life of the program. In most cases, this option is turned on during the validation phase of code development and then turned off during final production. In most cases, SYMBOLGEN does not add any additional information than that provided by MPRINT, but in cases like Example 4.14, SYMBOLGEN does add significant value to the validation process.

4.2.3.3 Using MLOGIC

Another SAS option that is very useful for validating and debugging complex macro code is MLOGIC. Again, this option produces many extra lines in the log so it is often only turned on during the validation process and turned off during production. It is also most useful when working with complex macro logic that directly affects what code is submitted to the SAS compiler (and hence MPRINT does not show evidence of the macro compilation). When you are using the same code as Example 4.14, the MLOGIC option shows the following in the log:

Output 4.15

```
538           %dostuff(invar=pr,cutoff=100)
MLOGIC(DOSTUFF):  Beginning execution.
MLOGIC(DOSTUFF):  Parameter INVAR has value pr
MLOGIC(DOSTUFF):  Parameter CUTOFF has value 100
MPRINT(DOSTUFF):   data dpr dropped;
MPRINT(DOSTUFF):   set vitals;
MPRINT(DOSTUFF):   by inv_no patid;
MPRINT(DOSTUFF):   retain prflag;
MPRINT(DOSTUFF):   if first.patid then prflag = .;
MPRINT(DOSTUFF):   if pr lt 100 and prflag lt 2 then prflag = 1;
MPRINT(DOSTUFF):   else if pr ge 100 then prflag = 2;
MPRINT(DOSTUFF):   if not last.patid then output dropped;
MPRINT(DOSTUFF):   else output dpr;
MPRINT(DOSTUFF):   run;

NOTE: There were 1727 observations read from the data set
      WORK.VITALS.
NOTE: The data set WORK.DPR has 244 observations and 19 variables.
NOTE: The data set WORK.DROPPED has 1483 observations and 19
      variables.
NOTE: DATA statement used (Total process time):
      real time           0.01 seconds
      cpu time            0.01 seconds


MLOGIC(DOSTUFF):  %IF condition &valid=1 is FALSE
MLOGIC(DOSTUFF):  Ending execution.
```

Notice how the bold row differs from the note produced by the SYMBOLGEN option. In this case, not only does MLOGIC list the value to which macro variable &VALID resolves, but it also reports how the macro compiler resolved the logical IF statement (in this case, FALSE). While this is a very simple example, it is easy to imagine how this option could facilitate the validation and debugging of macro code with more complex logic.

4.3 Techniques That Facilitate Validation

As with any tool, the tools that SAS provides to perform tasks are only effective if you use them well. When developing programs that must be validated, you must use all of the tools SAS provides to your best advantage.

4.3.1 Start with a Clean Log

One of the most important and simplest steps to making validation easier is to start with a clean log. This means that your log should not only be free of errors, but it should also be free of warnings and "helpful" notes. Helpful notes are notes in your log that let you know where SAS was trying to be helpful. These include notes like the following:

- NOTE: Numeric values have been converted to character values at the places given by: (Line):(Column).

- NOTE: Character values have been converted to numeric values at the places given by: (Line):(Column).

Other notes that describe problems with the data and/or how you are trying to process it should also be eliminated from the log. While these issues will not stop SAS from processing, they need to be addressed.

- NOTE: Invalid numeric data, VARNAME = value, at line XXX column NN.

- NOTE: Missing values were generated as a result of performing an operation on missing values.

- NOTE: MERGE statement has more than one data set with repeats of BY values.

- NOTE: Variable TEST is uninitialized.

If you start with a clean log that is free from all messages that could indicate an issue, it is much easier to notice real issues if they arise. Remember to review the entire log if the data has changed; don't just skip to the bottom of the program to look for fatal errors. If you start with a clean log, any issues caused by new data are easy to see as you quickly skim through the file. In addition, because the log is the easiest place to look for evidence of problems, this is usually the first place outside reviewers will look. An issue-free log can be the first step to gaining a reviewer's confidence in your work.

4.3.2 Print Only What You Need—When You Need It

Although PROC PRINT can be incredibly useful, it can also be misused. Printing data set after data set throughout the course of your program really doesn't add value to your validation effort. One of the best ways to ensure that the program is working as expected is by generating simple prints of selected *subsets* of records throughout the programming process. As discussed earlier in the chapter with PROC PRINT, the macro language can help you to easily select a specific subset of observations for review with simple macro assignments.

At the top of your program, set a macro variable to the subset of records you'd like to monitor throughout your program. When printing interim data sets, refer to this macro variable and you'll print the same subset of subjects. Placing this subset into a macro variable means the subset needs to be changed only once to affect the entire program. Recall the previous example:

Example 4.15

```
%let valpats=patid in(1 3 8);
proc print data = start (where=(&valpats));
   title "INCOMING DATA";
run;
…code that manipulates the data…
proc print data = middle (where=(&valpats));
   title "DATA AFTER MANIPULATION";
run;
```

If you notice potential data issues with other subjects, it's easy to add or remove subjects from the list of subjects in the &VALPATS macro variable. The next time you run your program, the new subset of records will print throughout. This simplifies the process of ensuring that your code handles the suspect data appropriately.

It is also important to distinguish between the code needed to validate programs that are being developed and the code needed to validate final production. A program must be checked at every step during development. However, when validation is finished and the programs are ready to produce official output, you will want to see validation printouts only for actual problems (not just for informational checking). Again, macros can simplify this process. Macros can be used to easily turn off output when switching between development and production without having to delete the actual code (it may be useful later if issues arise). One of the easiest ways to do this is to take advantage of the true/false logic in SAS. Consider the following code:

Example 4.16

```
%let printme = 1;
proc print data=orglib.demo (where=(&printme));
    title "INCOMING DEMO DATA";
run;
```

In this case, printing is simply informational (the code prints all records, not specific data issues). Because &PRINTME resolves to 1, which is always true, all of the records in the DEMO data set print (and a message from SAS is printed in your log WHERE 1 /* an obviously TRUE where clause */). When you no longer need to print these records, simply change the value of &PRINTME to 0 at the top of your program and no records will print because 0 is always false (again, SAS comments that WHERE 0 /* an obviously FALSE where clause */).

4.3.3 Tracking Problems

Most programmers do not start with perfect data. Even if the group that gave you the data insists that it has no problems, usually a few emerge in the course of merging and manipulating it for analysis purposes. As a programmer, you must be aware of any of these issues and deal with them effectively rather than allowing SAS to handle issues automatically.

4.3.3.1 Problem Data Sets

Whenever possible, use DATA steps rather than PROC SQL to combine data, so validation checks can be programmed to output to problem data sets. When merging, you should make sure that the data combines as intended. As demonstrated in the previous sections, even a simple merge between two data sets can have unexpected results that do not create syntax errors. Unless you check the log and then force a check to be performed, you probably would not know there was a problem. If you program in a little extra check using the IN= option, the program can almost monitor itself. A good example of using this option appeared in the code example we saw earlier in this chapter:

Example 4.17

```
data vitals checkme;
    merge vitals(in=invl)
          visit (in=invt);
    by inv_no patid visit;
    if invl and invt then output vitals;
                     else output checkme;
run;
```

When looking at the data for a study, you would expect that any data set record would be associated with a study visit. For the study data in this example, the visit dates are stored in a separate data set while all other data sets contain only a visit label. Each data set in the study should have a corresponding record in the VISIT data set (i.e., every visit should have a date associated with it), but this is not always true. When this code runs, the log shows that three records in the VITALS data set do not have a corresponding record in VISIT. Sending these three problem records to a data set makes the problem easier to find than it would be by just reviewing the log. These records are easily printed for further review. Without printing them, the program would report no errors, making it much more difficult to investigate the issue.

4.3.3.2 Flagging Problem Data

When you are working with the values within a data set, if data does not have the values you were expecting (you expect to see only a 1 or 0 value for a variable, but the data also has values of 9) or values do not occur in combinations you were expecting (a diagnostic test was performed, but no unit of measurement was provided), you can set a flagging variable to a value and then print the records with those values for review. Problem flags are also useful when you are trying to track how data is moving through complicated logic statements. Using these flags shows where a given data point falls in the logic you are moving through. The following code shows simplified examples of this technique:

Example 4.18

```
data flags;
    set orglib.vitals;
    if temp lt 96 or temp gt 104 then tcheck = 1;
    if pr gt 95 then
    do;
        gothere = 1;
        if resp le 16 then
        do;
            gothere = 2;
            if temp ge 99 then newvar = 1;
        end;
    end;
run;

proc print data=flags (where=(tcheck eq 1));
    var inv_no patid visit temp;
    title 'CHECK TEMPERATURE - DATA LOOKS TOO HIGH OR TOO LOW';
run;
```

```
proc print data=flags (where=(gothere ne .));
   var inv_no patid visit pr resp temp gothere newvar;
   title "CHECK LOGIC FOR NEWVAR";
run;
```

The first IF statement checks for data that is outside the expected range of results. The second IF statement begins a more complicated series of nested DO loops. This is a simple example, but more complicated logic could quickly become confusing and difficult to check. Adding the GOTHERE flag to a record makes it easy to check that the logic is working correctly. The results from each check are listed here:

Output 4.16

```
CHECK TEMPERATURE - DATA LOOKS TOO HIGH OR TOO LOW

Obs     INV_NO      PATID      VISIT        TEMP

   4        1          1      Week 2         N
 293        1         41      Week 6       104.8
 584        2         60      Week 3        95.3
 722        2         79      Week 2         N
 727        2         80      Day -8         N
 832        2         94      Week 4         N
1413        3        136      Day -8        74.0
1514        3        240      Week 6         D
1543        4        143      Week 6         N
1625        4        154      Week 6         N


CHECK LOGIC FOR NEWVAR

Obs   INV_NO  PATID  VISIT     PR  RESP   TEMP   gothere  newvar

  69      1       9   Week 5   104   14   99.4      2        1
  72      1      10   Day -1    98   12   98.4      2        .
 127      1      17   Week 6    97   14   98.8      2        .
 285      1      40   Week 4    96   14   98.4      2        .
 293      1      41   Week 6   100   18  104.8      1        .
 600      2      62   Week 3   100   16   98.6      2        .
 601      2      62   Week 6    96   16   99.3      2        1
 625      2      65   Week 6    96   14   97.9      2        .
 677      2      73   Week 5    98   14   97.3      2        .
1223      2     210   Week 2    98   16   98.0      2        .
1332      3     125   Week 4    96   18   97.9      1        .
1376      3     131   Week 1   100   16   97.0      2        .
```

The first output shows that there are records with missing values as well at data with values outside the expected range. The second output displays how the GOTHERE variable flags data that falls through the DATA step logic. In both cases, the code itself helps to check the data so all you need to do is review the problem cases rather than pages of printouts trying to pick out patterns or issues.

4.3.4 Using PROC TRANSPOSE or an Alternative Solution

It is not uncommon for clinical trial data to be collected in a structure that, while appropriate for data collection, is not ideal for data analysis. In these cases, it is often necessary to transpose the data from one layout to another, such as from one record per visit to one record per test so that you can calculate the change in result from visit to visit. SAS has provided a great tool in PROC TRANSPOSE for accomplishing this task. However, sometimes it is more appropriate to flip the data structure through DATA step processing rather than through PROC TRANSPOSE. In cases where you need to transpose with an ID statement, you must ensure that the ID variable has a value for every record; otherwise, some records will be dropped from the final data set. Consider the following example:

Example 4.19

```
proc transpose data=vitals out=tresp;
   by inv_no patid;
   id visit;
   var resp;
run;
```

In this example, the data set starts with one record per cycle and the resulting data set has one record per patient ID. Both the log and a partial print of the data before and after the transposition demonstrate how some of the data was dropped from the final data set.

The log results from PROC TRANSPOSE in Example 4.19 are shown in Output 4.17.

Output 4.17

```
359        proc transpose data=vitals out=tresp;
360           by inv_no patid;
361           id visit;
362           var resp;
363        run;
```

WARNING: 2 observations omitted due to missing ID values.
NOTE: There were 1727 observations read from the data set
      WORK.VITALS.
NOTE: The data set WORK.TRESP has 244 observations and 12 variables.
NOTE: PROCEDURE TRANSPOSE used (Total process time):
      real time   0.03 seconds
      cpu time   0.03 seconds

A print of 10 observations before and after the transposition is shown in Output 4.18.

Output 4.18

```
VITALS BEFORE TRANSPOSE

  Obs      INV_NO      PATID      VISIT      RESP

   1          1          1      Day -1        14
   2          1          1      Day -8        16
   3          1          1      Week 1        14
   4          1          1      Week 2         N
   5          1          1      Week 3        14
   6          1          1      Week 6        14
   7          1          2      Day -1        14
   8          1          2      Day -8        12
   9          1          2      Week 1        12
  10          1          2      Week 2        12

VITALS AFTER TRANSPOSE
```

	I		_	L		D	D	W	W	W	W	W	W
	N	P	N	A		a	a	e	e	e	e	e	e
	V	A	A	B		y	y	e	e	e	e	e	e
O	_	T	M	E		_	_	k	k	k	k	k	k
b	N	I	E	L		_	_	_	_	_	_	_	_
s	O	D	_	_		1	8	1	2	3	6	4	5

(continued)

```
 1   1    1   RESP   Respirations   14   16   14    N   14   14    .    .
 2   1    2   RESP   Respirations   14   12   12   12   12   12   12   12
 3   1    3   RESP   Respirations   14   16   16   14   14   14   16   14
 4   1    4   RESP   Respirations   16   16   16   14   14   14   14   14
 5   1    5   RESP   Respirations   14   14   12   12   12   12   14   12
 6   1    6   RESP   Respirations   12   12   14   14   14   14   12   14
 7   1    7   RESP   Respirations   14   14   16   16   14   14   16   14
 8   1    8   RESP   Respirations   14   14   16   14   14   14   16   14
 9   1    9   RESP   Respirations   12   12   14   14   16   16   14   14
10   1   10   RESP   Respirations   12   12   12   14   14   12   12   12
```

Notice that while a warning message in the log alerts you to this issue, there is no way to know which two records were omitted. The result might be correct, but there is no way to be sure. Don't ignore this warning. The code will not pass the final validation step with a warning in the log.

There are several methods to work around this issue (for example, filter these problem records out before sending the data through PROC TRANSPOSE). The key is that PROC TRANSPOSE makes some assumptions about the data and you need to ensure that those assumptions are correct before executing it.

You can also transpose data using the DATA step. One alternative method to using PROC TRANSPOSE—merging data to itself—was discussed earlier in the chapter. The DATA step can be used in other ways to transpose data using arrays and retained variables. While using the DATA step is a longer, more manual approach, it does have advantages. First, a DATA step offers all of the techniques presented earlier in this chapter to check the data and make sure it meets any assumptions. Second, if the data needs to be manipulated with a DATA step so that PROC TRANSPOSE works correctly (to combine variables or filter records), the data can be transposed with the DATA step itself. To make the transposition in Example 4.20 work correctly, you'll need to

1. remove records with missing visit IDs

2. sort the data

3. execute PROC TRANSPOSE

Alternately, you could sort the data and then transpose it in the DATA step. Consider the following:

Example 4.20

```
data dresp (keep=inv_no patid visit test diff day: week:)
    check (keep=inv_no patid visit barcode);
  set vitals;
  by inv_no patid visit;

  ** CHECK FOR BAD ID VALUES **;
  if compress(visit) eq ' ' then output check;

  ** SET UP FOR TRANSPOSE **;
  retain day_8 day_1 week1 - week6;
  array vars {8} day_8 day_1 week1 - week6;
  array tpts {8} $12 _temporary_ ('DAY -8' 'DAY -1' 'WEEK 1' 'WEEK 2'
                                  'WEEK 3' 'WEEK 4' 'WEEK 5' 'WEEK 6');
  ** RESET TEMP VARS FOR EACH NEW PATIENT **;
  if first.patid then
  do i = 1 to 8;
     vars{i} = .;
  end;
  ** FILL IN VARS HOLDING TRANSPOSED DATA **;
  do i = 1 to 8;
     test = "RESP";
     if upcase(visit) eq tpts{i} then vars{i} = resp;
  end;
  ** CALCULATE END OF STUDY CHANGE FROM BASELINE AND OUTPUT **;
  if last.patid then
  do;
     if nmiss(day_1, week6) eq 0 then diff = week6 - day_1;
     output dresp;
  end;
run;
proc print data=check;
  title 'PROBLEM: MISSING VISIT ID';
run;
```

Although this code is longer and more complicated, it offers a few advantages. It handles cases where VISIT is missing without any warning messages in the log, it checks for data issues and prints any that are found, and it calculates a new variable. All of this is accomplished in one pass through the data set. So, while on the surface this code may take a little longer to produce, you can program in data and logic checks that may save time over the course of the project. The main point to these examples is that there are two methods for transposing data and you should consider the pros and cons of each when deciding which to use in a given situation.

4.3.5 Tracking Dropped Data

There are often cases where data has extra records that need to be removed. Sometimes these are records that have missing data and, therefore, are not useful. Some records may be created in the process of calculating new information, and others may contain data that is unnecessary for the task you want to perform. Regardless of the reason, these records should not be deleted without confirming that they are the records you expect.

4.3.5.1 Don't Delete

Often you might want to remove unnecessary records from a data set. For example, you might not want to keep records with missing values for select variables. It is often tempting to code a simple statement like if temp lt 0 then delete; and move on. Unfortunately, this does not allow you to check that the deleted records are the ones you intended. Instead, consider the code and output below:

Example 4.21

```
data temp dropped;
    set vitals (keep=inv_no patid visit temp);
    if temp lt 0 then output dropped;
                else output temp;
run;

proc print data=dropped;
    title 'TEMP LESS THAN 0 SO DROPPED FROM DATA SET';
run;
```

Output 4.19

```
421          data temp dropped;
422             set vitals (keep=inv_no patid visit temp);
423             if temp lt 0 then output dropped;
424                         else output temp;
425          run;

NOTE: There were 1727 observations read from the data set
      WORK.VITALS.
NOTE: The data set WORK.TEMP has 1720 observations and 4 variables.
NOTE: The data set WORK.DROPPED has 7 observations and 4 variables.
NOTE: DATA statement used (Total process time):
      real time              0.01 seconds
      cpu time               0.01 seconds
```

Output 4.20 displays the records that were dropped from the data set. Note that two values were actually dropped—two different special missing values (.N and .D). While this result is probably acceptable, deleting the records would not have shown that the data being dropped encompassed more than simple missing values.

Output 4.20

```
TEMP LESS THAN 0 SO DROPPED FROM DATA SET

Obs      PATID     INV_NO     VISIT        TEMP

 1          1         1       Week 2         N
 2         79         2       Week 2         N
 3         80         2       Day -8         N
 4         94         2       Week 4         N
 5        240         3       Week 6         D
 6        143         4       Week 6         N
 7        154         4       Week 6         N
```

4.3.5.2 Drop Your Own Duplicates

Often data sets contain duplicate records that need to be removed. These duplicates can come from a variety of sources. Often it is simply a matter of counting the right records. For example, a patient may have had a high temperature four different times over the duration of the trial, but you only need to know if the patient *ever* had a high temperature. To get an accurate count, only one record is needed per patient. All of the rest would contain duplicate information.

There are two methods to remove these extra records. One way is with PROC SORT and the NODUPKEY or NODUPREC option; the other is with a DATA step. As with most methods in SAS, one can be more appropriate than the other depending on the situation. Understanding each method's strengths can help you can decide which to use.

Before the release of SAS 9, using the DATA step was the only way to drop duplicate records and retain the ability to see which records were dropped. While there are other options with SAS 9, this method still has merit because the DATA step can handle multiple tasks at the same time that duplicate records are being removed. Consider the following code, where observations with duplicate information are dropped and a flag indicating severity of abnormality is also created:

Example 4.22

```
data dtemp dropped;
   set vitals (where=(pr gt 90));
   by inv_no patid;
   retain sevflag;
   if first.patid then sevflag = .;
        if pr lt 100 and sevflag lt 2 then sevflag = 1;
   else if pr ge 100                   then sevflag = 2;
   if not last.patid then output dropped;
                    else output dtemp;
run;
proc print data=dtemp (obs=20);
   var inv_no patid visit pr sevflag;
   title 'PATIENTS WITH HEART RATE OVER 90 WITH SEVERITY FLAG';
run;
proc print data=dropped;
   var inv_no patid visit pr sevflag;
   title 'DUPLICATES DROPPED - CHECK SEVERITY FLAG';
run;
```

Output 4.21

```
PATIENTS WITH HEART RATE OVER 90 WITH SEVERITY FLAG (10 OBS)

Obs     INV_NO     PATID     VISIT       PR     sevflag

  1        1          8      Week 5      93        1
  2        1          9      Week 5     104        2
  3        1         10      Day -1      98        1
  4        1         17      Week 6      97        1
  5        1         40      Week 4      96        1
  6        1         41      Week 6     100        2
  7        1        187      Day -1      92        1
  8        1        190      Week 2      94        1
  9        1        195      Week 6      93        1
 10        1        198      Week 2      94        1
```

(continued)

```
DUPLICATES DROPPED - CHECK SEVERITY FLAG

Obs      INV_NO      PATID      VISIT       PR      sevflag

  1         1           8       Day  -1      93         1
  2         1          41       Week  1      91         1
  3         2          44       Day  -1      92         1
  4         2          62       Week  3     100         2
  5         2         207       Week  1     100         2
  6         2         210       Day  -1      96         1
  7         2         210       Day  -8     100         2
  8         3         119       Day  -8      92         1
  9         3         125       Week  1      92         1
 10         4         149       Day  -1      96         1
```

This output indicates that the correct records are being dropped from the final data set.

SAS 9 also added the DUPOUT= option to PROC SORT. This option puts any duplicate records that are dropped with the NODUPKEY or NODUPREC options into a separate data set. The DUPOUT= option was a huge improvement for validation. Prior to the addition of this option, only the DATA step allowed you to drop duplicate records and still be able to check what was dropped. Now, programmers can use the easy functionality of PROC SORT and still check which records were dropped from the main data set. The code below shows the results of using the DUPOUT= option:

Example 4.23

```
proc sort data=vitals (where=(pr gt 90))
             out=htemp  nodupkey dupout=dropped;
   by inv_no patid;
run;
proc print data=htemp (obs=10);
   var inv_no patid visit pr;
   title '10 OBS OF PATIENTS WITH PULSE RATE OVER 90';
run;
proc print data=dropped;
   var inv_no patid visit pr;
   title 'DUPLICATES DROPPED FROM PROC SORT';
run;
```

Output 4.22

```
10 OBS OF PATIENTS WITH PULSE RATE OVER 90

Obs      INV_NO      PATID      VISIT        PR

  1         1           8       Day -1       93
  2         1           9       Week 5      104
  3         1          10       Day -1       98
  4         1          17       Week 6       97
  5         1          40       Week 4       96
  6         1          41       Week 1       91
  7         1         187       Day -1       92
  8         1         190       Week 2       94
  9         1         195       Week 6       93
 10         1         198       Week 2       94


DUPLICATES DROPPED FROM PROC SORT

Obs      INV_NO      PATID      VISIT        PR

  1         1           8       Week 5       93
  2         1          41       Week 6      100
  3         2          44       Week 1       92
  4         2          62       Week 6       96
  5         2         207       Week 2      100
  6         2         210       Day -8      100
  7         2         210       Week 2       98
  8         3         119       Week 1       92
  9         3         125       Week 4       96
 10         4         149       Day -8       96
```

Once again, it is obvious from this output that the dropped records are appropriate. This output proves that your syntax is working correctly. While this method involves much less code than the DATA step method, you would still need to use a DATA step to add the severity flag to this data. The DATA step is still used frequently to remove duplicates because multiple tasks can be accomplished in one step.

4.4 Conclusion

Many of the techniques discussed in this chapter can be used for many tasks, regardless of the type of data being referenced. In addition to simply knowing the general techniques, you need to understand how and when to apply them. Knowing *what* to look for is critical, while knowing *how* to look for it can always be learned. There are also more specific validation tasks that apply to the type of data being manipulated or to the task being performed. In the following chapters, we explore the validation considerations for the more common tasks and types of data encountered in clinical trials.

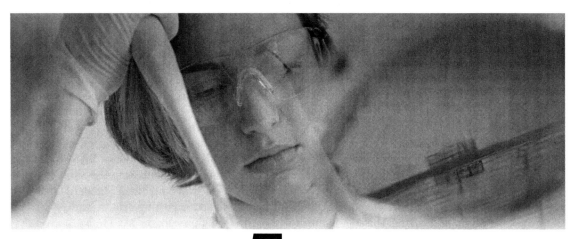

Chapter 5

Data Import and Export

5.1 Introduction

Although the majority of study data is collected via a Case Report form (CRF), that data can reach a programmer from a variety of sources. Different database software systems can be used to house the CRF data, and some data collected for the study might not be captured on the CRF. For example, clinical laboratory data is often analyzed by a central laboratory, and the results of the analysis are transferred directly from the lab to the group holding the CRF database. In the end, regardless of the original source and format of the data, it is all eventually converted to SAS data sets for final reporting purposes. In most cases, it is a SAS programmer's responsibility to get this data into or out of SAS. When transforming data, simply using an import or export wizard and checking for errors in the log is not sufficient. Typically, companies will develop and maintain Standard Operating Procedures (SOPs) and guidelines for importing and exporting data, regardless of the origin of the data. These guidelines will outline what procedures need to be followed to ensure that any transfer of data occurs accurately. In this area more than perhaps any other, the validation process is critical. If the data underlying an analysis cannot be proven correct, that analysis is worthless. Because data might be collected in many places and transferred from one software package to another as well as one location to another, there are many places where validation comes into play. This chapter discusses many of the items to check for when validating data that is transferred to and imported from various sources.

5.2 Validating the Import Process

Data can be sent to the programming group from a variety of sources, including an internal data management group or an external third party such as a clinical laboratory or electrocardiogram (ECG) analysis lab. Regardless of the source of the data, it is important to understand what is being sent and how. Obtaining this information can be one of the most frustrating pieces of the validation process for programmers. Because programmers are on the receiving end of the data, they often have little control over how much information they are sent as documentation with the data. Ideally, a format for both the data and its documentation would be agreed upon between the group sending the data and the programmers receiving it prior to the first transfer of data. The items that are documented should be similar to those you would expect to provide if you were sending files rather than receiving them. These items include the following:

- File format of the data being sent (SAS data set, SAS transport file, ASCII file, Microsoft Excel spreadsheet, other?)

- Amount of data being sent (cumulative data or only data that is new or updated since the previous transfer?)

- Structure of the data being sent (variable names, types, expected values; number of records per subject, visit, etc.)

- If the data is supporting the CRF database (for example, clinical lab data), the information that is common between the CRF database and the supporting data (will both have the same subject identifiers, visit labels, or other identifying fields?)

- The number of records being sent with each transfer, especially if the data being sent is not a SAS file

Depending on the source of the data (internal or external) and its file type (SAS file or other), the task of validating that the data being imported is what was intended will vary in difficulty. Regardless of the data being imported, it is critical to document what was done to the data and that the result was validated against any attending documentation, as well as any other related data in the database.

Although the SAS Import Wizard can easily convert data from another file format into SAS data sets, for validation purposes it is important that a program be generated and stored, along with the log and any validation output created by that import program. Ideally, import programs (and any validation output they generate) should be written and stored in their own location with their own naming conventions. In this way, if any imported data is suspect, you can check these files to ensure that the import process was done correctly. For the same reason, it is also important to keep import programs as simple as possible. These programs should only import the data and create any output needed to validate the import process and the data imported. Removing extraneous variables or records, merging with other data sets, or other tasks should be done in separate programs. While adding to the data is not recommended, it is often necessary during the validation process to ensure that the data itself (beyond the structure) is what is expected—not just for one transfer but across transfers as the study continues. For these reasons, the following procedures are recommended when importing data:

- Create and maintain an archive area in which older versions of the data and the program used for import and validation can reside. This archive will enable anyone to compare different versions of the data at any time. This area should be created at the beginning of data capture and maintained throughout the course of a study. The import archive area should be a separate location than that which houses the working copy of the data.

- Request from the sender copies of the PROC CONTENTS and PROC PRINT output for the data being sent (or the equivalent information for file formats that are not specific to SAS). After the data has been imported, a comparison of these documents to the PROC CONTENTS and PROC PRINT output from the imported data can be done and kept as evidence of validation.

- If the data being sent is only a subset of a larger database (for example, ECG results), be sure to compare key identifiers in the subset data to the main database. There should not be records for subjects in the subset data that do not exist in the main clinical database; the reverse might also be true. Depending on the structure of the data subset, other variables (such as age or sex) might also need to be reconciled.

- For data that is sent more than once, it is good practice to compare the current data against earlier versions to ensure that the current data changes are accurate and expected. In some cases you may only need to compare data structures, but in others you may need to compare the content as well. Using PROC COMPARE to do this is discussed later in this chapter.

5.3 Validating the Export Process

The export process is perhaps the easier of the two data exchange processes to validate. In exporting data, the programmer has complete knowledge of the data being sent and total control of the process followed to generate the file(s) being exported. Again, although the SAS Export Wizard can generate a number of different file types from SAS data sets, in the clinical trial world it is critical not only to be able to prove that what was done was correct, but also to be able to reliably reproduce the same results. Both of these requirements mean that a program must be stored and the log and output reviewed. In addition, documentation detailing the requirements for the data transfer is essential.

There are many details that programmers need to know to complete and validate a data transfer successfully. These include, but are not limited to, the following:

- Data to be transferred (all data in the CRF database or some subset?)

- Structure of the data to be transferred (is the data as it is currently stored adequate, or will the data need additional or fewer variables, will data from different data sets need to be combined, or will some other form of data manipulation need to be done before sending?)

- File format to transfer (SAS data sets, SAS transport files, Excel worksheets, other?)

- Method of transfer (via e-mail in a password-protected zip file, CD via courier, other?)

- Recipient of the data (client, consultant, other?)

Each of these pieces of information must be documented thoroughly so that once a data transfer is prepared and ready for export, a second person can validate the transfer. In the end, another programmer should be able to start with the same data, apply the specifications, and get the same resulting files as were originally sent. It is not uncommon for recipients of data to ask for the same data to be sent again, often much later than the original transfer. This could be for a variety of reasons: the original data might have been sent via CD and that CD was lost, or the data might need to be sent to an additional recipient and needs to be sent from a source that can validate the transfer. Regardless of the reason, programmers must assume that data transfers must be reproducible at any time. In addition, with the rising prevalence of Clinical Research Organizations (CROs) in the clinical development process, the FDA does pay particular attention to the traceability of data. This makes the documentation and validation of data transfers even more critical.

5.4 General Items to Watch For When Transferring Data

As you gain more experience with the import and export of data, you will learn what types of issues to look for when checking the data resulting from any import or export processing you perform. Issues surrounding some of the more common data types encountered with data transfers are discussed in more detail later. The following are a few of the more common issues you will need to consider, regardless of file type and whether data is being imported or exported:

- Date issues—make sure all dates are imported or exported correctly. The importance of this issue depends on the file type you are working with, but in general you need to make sure that this type of data is handled correctly.

- Data types—the default number of rows SAS reviews when deciding what type of data is in a column is only 20 rows. When importing data from a file type other than SAS, if you let SAS decide on the data type stored in a column, make sure that all the data is of the same type (i.e., no mixed data types). If you see missing values in a numeric variable, make sure the data was truly missing and not a character value that got lost during the import process. Consider using the GUESSINGROWS option on PROC IMPORT so that SAS will check a larger number of values to identify the type. When exporting data, make sure the data type meets any specifications that you are working from (the SAS data sets may have stored the data as a numeric variable, but you may need to export that same data as a character field).

- Truncation—as a default, SAS reviews only 20 rows when deciding the length needed for a character variable. Make sure you review text values to make sure no values are truncated (find the longest value in the imported file for each text variable and check those records in your new data). If you specify variable widths when exporting data, make sure those widths are wide enough to accommodate the largest text value in the data.

- File content—if you are "manually" importing or exporting data (via a program rather than a wizard), make sure all of the variables from the original file are included in the new one. Also, if you import or export the data more than once with the same program, make sure the structure of the original data hasn't changed (variables weren't added or removed that your program doesn't account for).

Regardless of file type or whether data is being imported or exported, the validation process should always contain two basic goals:

1. Ensure that the resulting data accurately represents the original data.

2. Ensure that the resulting data matches the specifications provided. How those two goals are accomplished will vary depending on the file type and whether the data is being imported or exported.

In all cases, it is important to document the process followed and the results of all validation efforts.

5.5 Working with SAS Files

SAS files are the easiest to work with for programmers for a variety of reasons. It is often easy to get and create information about this type of data via PROC CONTENTS and other procedures such as PROC PRINT and PROC FREQ. Although this type of data is easy to work with, there are still validation steps that must be performed to ensure that the data being sent or received is what was intended.

5.5.1 SAS Data Sets

While SAS data sets do not appear to require any validation (you can simply copy them from one place to another via Windows Explorer), it is recommended that the data sets first be placed in a separate area for review before copying them to their final destination. The data should be validated before it updates or replaces existing data to make sure that there are no problems. Two common problems that must be addressed are incompatible SAS versions and the existence of attached user-defined formats.

The versions of SAS used to create and import a data set might be different, and programmers cannot assume that all SAS users are using the most current release. For example, data sets sent from an external source might have the file extension .SD2 (a SAS 6 data set). If the main data library is SAS 9, you might need to convert the SAS 6 files to SAS

9 before adding the new data to the main library. In addition, files with the .SAS7BDAT extension could have been created either with SAS 8 or SAS 9. Reviewing the output from PROC CONTENTS is the only way to verify which version of SAS was used to create the data. While importing data from different versions of SAS might not create any problems, unexpected issues could arise. It is important to be aware of potential issues and to verify that none occurred during processing.

The other important piece of information to understand about a data set is whether or not user-defined formats are stored with the permanent data set. If data is stored with user-defined formats attached, having the format catalog (or a program that will create it) is just as important as having the data itself. While it is always preferable to have the format catalog in these cases, if a catalog cannot be provided or created, it might be necessary to remove these user-defined formats for programs to be run without error (a simple FORMAT _ALL_; statement in a DATA step will do this). If formats are attached and the appropriate catalog cannot be provided, the NOFMTERR option can be used; however, this option might not be appropriate for all data sets in a library. Rather than turning off a SAS option that is helpful for the validation of other tasks, it is often safer simply to "disconnect" formats that do not exist. If you are sending data to an external client and user-defined formats are attached to the data sets, be sure to include both the format catalog and the program that created it. If the recipient of the data is working with a different version of SAS, or on a different platform, they might need to re-create the catalog for it to work properly.

Whether importing or exporting data as SAS data sets, it is important to verify what version of SAS is being used and whether user-defined formats are stored with the data sets. When importing SAS data sets, there might be an additional step to the validation process, beyond confirming that the PROC CONTENTS output from the data received matches the documentation sent with the data. If the data being received is only a small part of a larger clinical database, you might need to validate the actual content of the data set(s) as mentioned earlier in the chapter.

5.5.2 SAS Transport Files

Transport files are the file type of choice for sending data to the FDA. Likewise, they are generally the file type of choice for programmers to receive. There are several items to keep in mind when validating files sent in this format. First and most critical, transport files can be created two different ways—via PROC COPY and via PROC CPORT. In both cases, the file extension is determined by the user and not the procedure that created the file. So, although the general convention for naming transport files is FILENAME.XPT, there is no way to know by looking at the filename whether this file 1) contains many data sets or only one data set, or 2) whether the file was created with PROC COPY or PROC CPORT. When exporting data in this file format, unless the recipient specifically requests that the data be sent through PROC CPORT, the default method of creation should be with PROC COPY. When receiving data from an outside source, it is important to ask how the transport files are being created. If possible, request that they be generated with PROC COPY.

Another item to keep in mind is that the FDA requires that each data set be in its own transport file and that those files be created with PROC COPY. However, for other data transfers, it is possible to include all data sets in a library in a single transport file. It is important to understand what is included in the transport file so that the proper import methods, archival preparations, and validation steps can be put in place and executed effectively.

5.6 Working with Other File Types

In addition to SAS file formats, other file formats, such as Microsoft Excel and simple ASCII files, are often used to transfer data between sources. Whereas importing and exporting data in SAS file formats gives programmers access to many SAS tools for programmatic validation of data transfers (such as PROC CONTENTS and PROC COMPARE), other software packages do not have similar tools. As a result, importing or exporting data in other file types involves more manual activities, such as manual comparisons of output generated from each source.

5.6.1 Microsoft Excel Files

Although SAS makes exporting Microsoft Excel files simple, they are often some of the most complicated files to import, especially when those files are generated manually rather than programmatically. When exporting data as Excel files, there are generally two ways to validate that the Excel file accurately represents the SAS data set from which it was created. The first method involves creating an Excel file and then re-importing that file into a work data set and comparing the re-imported file to the original SAS data set. If these two match, then the Excel file is accurate. The second method involves generating PROC CONTENTS output, PROC PRINT output for the first and last observations, frequencies of categorical data, and simple statistics for continuous data. Once the SAS documentation is generated, the first and last observations are printed from the Excel file, as well as similar statistics for data. The output from each file is then manually compared. The size of the files (how many variables as well as how many records) dictates which method is more appropriate.

Importing data from Excel files can be tricky, particularly when the data was entered manually. Unlike SAS, Excel allows more than one data type within a single column. By default, SAS reads only the first 20 rows of a file to determine what type of data is contained in that column. If the first 20 rows contain numeric data, but the 25th row contains a character value, that value will not be imported accurately. Dates are especially critical to check. When reviewing Excel data, all of the data might appear to be the same, but some might be formatted numeric values, while others might be character values. For this reason, it is critical to check the log from the import program for any unusual messages, run all categorical data through PROC FREQ, and manually review the content of the Excel file against selected printouts of the SAS data set to ensure that the data was imported as expected. Occasionally, importing data accurately requires that you save Excel data to another intermediate file type such as a CSV file or tab-delimited text file (both file types are available from within Excel). In these cases, it is important to use the original Excel file when validating the SAS data set that is created.

Because of the amount of data captured and transferred in Excel, it is worthwhile for SAS programmers to become familiar with this software package. Understanding how to generate frequency counts, sums, and means within Excel can help tremendously in the validation process. By knowing how to create output equivalent to that created by SAS, programmers can effectively validate data transfers quickly.

5.6.2 Flat Files

Flat (ASCII) files are another file format commonly used for transferring data. This file format allows for a variety of ways to store the data. Usually the data is stored either in fixed columns (for example, subject ID is always in columns 1 through 5, while sex is always in column 10) or with some delimiter between columns (such as a comma or pipe character). Whether importing or exporting data in this file format, it is critical to understand what the exact format and structure of the data should be. This information is used for creating programs to accurately transform the data, but more importantly for validation.

When exporting data in this format, the validation process includes making sure that the data is stored per specification as well as ensuring that the data was transformed accurately. Similar to working with Excel files, there are two methods used to validate the export of data as flat files. For larger data sets, it is often useful to export the flat file, re-import it into a work data set, and compare that to the original SAS file. In this case, it is important to make sure when re-importing the files that each variable's data type (character or numeric) is maintained so they can be compared accurately. Alternately, for smaller files with fewer variables, it might be simpler just to print out the resulting flat file and manually compare it to the original SAS data set.

Understanding the data structure when importing data in this format enables accurate importation of the data, and also enables validation that the content is complete (i.e., that no records or variables were omitted erroneously). Any notes in the log warning of lost cards or truncated values should be investigated and fixed. In addition to checking frequencies of categorical variables, it is also important to check that text field values are not truncated during import.

5.7 Common Procedures Used for Validating Data Transfers

The most commonly used SAS procedures for checking data are CONTENTS, PRINT, FREQ, MEANS (or UNIVARIATE), and COMPARE. Each of these procedures gives the programmer a unique look at the data in question. Depending on the size of the data set (5 observations or 5,000) and the type of data (categorical or continuous), each of these procedures is helpful to a different degree. Whereas we discussed ways to use PROC PRINT and PROC FREQ in Chapter 4, here we discuss efficient ways to use PROC CONTENTS and PROC COMPARE for validating the import or export of data.

5.7.1 PROC CONTENTS

This procedure is used to determine the structure and basic content of a data set. The most common use of the output is to see what variables are named, what type they are (character, numeric, date, time, etc.), and what the descriptive label says about what the variables contain. There are many more elements to PROC CONTENTS output that can be very useful when checking data.

The POSITION option on the PROC CONTENTS statement reports variables in the order in which they occur in the data set, in addition to the standard alphabetical order. This can be helpful if your data requirements dictate the order of the variables in your data set. This is often the case when data is being sent to an external source; when viewing the data it is often helpful to have the ID variables occur first. The following example demonstrates the output produced with the POSITION option. Note that this option gives output in addition to the standard alphabetical variable list, not in place of it. If you only want the list of variables in position order, the VARNUM option in SAS 9 will produce this list instead of the alphabetical list.

Example 5.1

```
libname sublib 'C:\Book\Examples\Data\Submission' ;
proc contents data=sublib.demo position ;
   title "CONTENTS OF DEMOGRAPHY DATA SET WITH POSITION STATEMENT" ;
run ;
```

Output 5.1 First variable list—alphabetical order

```
        CONTENTS OF DEMOGRAPHY DATA SET WITH POSITION STATEMENT

                      The CONTENTS Procedure

Data Set Name: SUBLIB.DEMO              Observations:         244
Member Type:   DATA                     Variables:            29
Engine:        V8                       Indexes:              0
Created:       11:10 Monday, October    Observation Length:   224
               13, 2003
Last Modified: 11:10 Monday, October    Deleted Observations: 0
               13, 2003
Protection:                             Compressed:           NO
Data Set Type:                          Sorted:               YES
Label:         Demographics


             -----Engine/Host Dependent Information-----

Data Set Page Size:          16384
Number of Data Set Pages:    4
First Data Page:             1
Max Obs per Page:            72
Obs in First Data Page:      53
Number of Data Set Repairs:  0
File Name:                   C:\Book\Examples\Data\Submission\
                             demo.sas7bdat
Release Created:             8.0202M0
Host Created:                WIN_PRO


             -----Alphabetic List of Variables and Attributes-----

  # Variable Type Len Pos Format     Informat   Label
----------------------------------------------------------------------
 20 BIRTHDT  Num    8  56 YYMMDD10.  MMDDYY10.  Date of Birth
  5 INV_NO   Num    8   0                       numeric siteid
                                                for merging
  6 SUBJID   Num    8   8                       numeric subjid
                                                for merging
 11 RACECD   Num    3 220                        race code
 12 RACEOTH  Char  30 156                        Race Specify
  9 GENDERCD Num    3 217                        Gender code
  8 SUBJINIT Char   3 147                        subject initials
 25 VISIT    Char   6 211                        visit name
```

(continued)

```
14 age      Num     8  16                      age in years
15 agegrpcd Num     8  24                      age group code
26 comply   Num     8  96                      1=has min compliance
                                               to be eff eval
 2 country  Char    3 139                       country
24 dmendt   Num     8  88 YYMMDD10.            study drug stop date
23 dmrefdt  Num     8  80 YYMMDD10.            study drug start date
16 height   Num     8  32                      height in centimeters
21 icdt     Num     8  64 YYMMDD10. MMDDYY10.  Date signed informed
                                               consent
29 pflageff Num     8 120                      1=efficacy population
28 pflagint Num     8 112                      1=intent-to-treat
                                               population
27 pflagsaf Num     8 104                      1=Safety population
13 race     Char   15 186                      race
22 randdt   Num     8  72 YYMMDD10. MMDDYY10.  Randomization date
 7 scrnid   Num     4 128                      Screening Number
10 sgender  Char    6 150                      Gender
 3 siteid   Char    2 142                      Site ID
 1 studyid  Char    7 132                      client protocol
                                               designation
 4 subjid   Char    3 144                      Subject ID
18 trtcd    Num     8  48                      treatment code
19 trtgrp   Char   10 201                      treatment group
17 weight   Num     8  40                      weight in kilograms
```

Output 5.2 Second variable list—position order

```
        CONTENTS OF DEMOGRAPHY DATA SET WITH POSITION STATEMENT

                       The CONTENTS Procedure

               -----Variables Ordered by Position-----

 # Variable Type Len Pos Format     Informat  Label
-----------------------------------------------------------------------
 1 studyid  Char   7 132                      client protocol
                                              designation
 2 country  Char   3 139                      country
 3 siteid   Char   2 142                      Site ID
 4 subjid   Char   3 144                      Subject ID
 5 INV_NO   Num    8   0                      numeric siteid
                                              for merging
```

(continued)

```
 6 SUBJID    Num    8   8                              numeric subjid
                                                       for merging
 7 scrnid    Num    4 128                              Screening Number
 8 SUBJINIT  Char   3 147                              subject initials
 9 GENDERCD  Num    3 217                              sex code
10 sgender   Char   6 150                              sex
11 RACECD    Num    3 220                              race code
12 RACEOTH   Char  30 156                              Race Specify
13 race      Char  15 186                              race
14 age       Num    8  16                              age in years
15 agegrpcd  Num    8  24                              age group code
16 height    Num    8  32                              height in centimeters
17 weight    Num    8  40                              weight in kilograms
18 trtcd     Num    8  48                              treatment code
19 trtgrp    Char  10 201                              treatment group
20 BIRTHDT   Num    8  56 YYMMDD10. MMDDYY10. Date of Birth
21 icdt      Num    8  64 YYMMDD10. MMDDYY10. Date signed informed
                                                       consent
22 randdt    Num    8  72 YYMMDD10. MMDDYY10. Randomization date
23 dmrefdt   Num    8  80 YYMMDD10.           study drug start date
24 dmendt    Num    8  88 YYMMDD10.           study drug stop date
25 VISIT     Char   6 211                              visit name
26 comply    Num    8  96                              1=has min compliance
                                                       to be eff eval
27 pflagsaf  Num    8 104                              1=Safety population
28 pflagint  Num    8 112                              1=intent-to-treat
                                                       population
29 pflageff  Num    8 120                              1=efficacy population
```

If the data set being reviewed was sorted when it was permanently stored (using PROC SORT or PROC SQL, for example), PROC CONTENTS also provides the sort information. Ideally, each data set is stored sorted by the variables required to identify a unique record.

Output 5.3 Sort Information from PROC CONTENTS

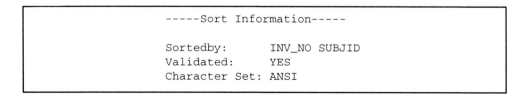

```
            -----Sort Information-----

      Sortedby:       INV_NO SUBJID
      Validated:      YES
      Character Set: ANSI
```

Overall, PROC CONTENTS provides a great deal of information about the structure of a data set. This can be used to validate that the data being transferred at least meets structural requirements and expectations.

5.7.2 PROC COMPARE

This procedure is invaluable when comparing previous data to current data, and also when comparing data transferred to a different file format as described earlier in the chapter. In addition to the usual comparisons between data sets, PROC COMPARE can be used in conjunction with PROC CONTENTS to compare the structure of data sets, which is especially useful when the actual content of the data sets is expected to change. Rather than manually checking to see if the new data is in the same structure as data previously received, create an output data set from PROC CONTENTS for both the new and old data sets, and then use PROC COMPARE to check that the structures are the same.

In the following example, ECG data was transferred from a central laboratory for inclusion in an analysis. The lab transferred draft data last month and final data this month. The structure of the data was expected to be the same for each transfer. Rather than simply importing the new data, running the analysis programs, and hoping for the best, we can use PROC CONTENTS and PROC COMPARE to check the data. Note that variables that are expected to differ between the two data sets are dropped before PROC COMPARE is run. These variables include the creation date, the last modified date, the library name, and the variable positions.

Example 5.2

```
proc contents data=onelib.ecg
              out =first (drop=crdate modate libname npos varnum)
              noprint ;
run ;


proc print data=first (obs=5) ;
   title "FIRST 5 OBS FROM CONTENTS DATA SET OF 1ST ECG DATA SEND" ;
run ;
```

Output 5.4 PROC PRINT output of data set created by PROC CONTENTS

```
       FIRST 5 OBS FROM CONTENTS DATA SET OF 1ST ECG DATA SEND


         M                                                    I
     M   E T                                              F F N I I
     E   M Y                    L                       F O O F N N
     M   L P                    E L                     O R R O F F
     N   A E N          T       N A                     R M M R O O
  O  A   B M A          Y       G B                     M A A M R R
  b  M   E E M          P       T E                     A T T A M M
  s  E   L M E          E       H L                     T L D T L D

  1 ECG      CONDUCT  2 200 CONDUCTION COMMENT                 0 0    0 0
  2 ECG      DATE_REC 1   8 DATE RECORDED              DATE 9 0        0 0
  3 ECG      HR       1   8 HEART RATE                         0 0    0 0
  4 ECG      HRN      1   8 NUMBER OF HR VALUES MEANED          0 0    0 0
  5 ECG      INTRP    2  20 INTERPRETATION                     0 0    0 0


                  I           I           C       S     N  N      P
                  D     M      D  P        O       O C C O   O  E  O       G
               E  D  X  E  X   R     M     S R H O D   D  N  I  G G E
               N  E  U  M  C   O  F  P  R  O T A L U   U  C  N  E E N
      J     N  G  L  S  T  O   T  L  R  E  R E R L P   P  R  T  N N N
  O   U     O  I  O  A  Y  U   E  A  E  U  T D S A K   R  Y  O  M N E
  b   S  B  N  B  G  P  N   C  G  S  S  E  B E T E   E  P  B  A U X
  s   T  S  E  S  E  E  T   T  S  S  E  D Y T E Y  C  T  S  X M T

  1 0 7579 V8 0 NONE DATA 0 --- --- NO NO . .     NO NO NO YES 0 . .
  2 1 7579 V8 0 NONE DATA 0 --- --- NO NO . .     NO NO NO YES 0 . .
  3 1 7579 V8 0 NONE DATA 0 --- --- NO NO . .     NO NO NO YES 0 . .
  4 1 7579 V8 0 NONE DATA 0 --- --- NO NO . .     NO NO NO YES 0 . .
  5 0 7579 V8 0 NONE DATA 0 --- --- NO NO . .     NO NO NO YES 0 . .
```

Now that we have printed the data set and begun the review, we must check to be sure that the structure of the new data set is that of the old version. We begin by bringing in the new data set into a WORK data set using PROC CONTENTS.

Example 5.3

```
proc contents data=twolib.ecg
          out =second (drop=crdate modate libname npos varnum)
          noprint ;
run ;
```

We now run the PROC COMPARE between the old data and the new:

Example 5.4

```
proc compare data=first compare=second listall ;
    id name ;
    title "COMPARE FIRST SEND TO SECOND SEND" ;
run ;
```

Output 5.5 Output from PROC COMPARE

```
               COMPARE FIRST SEND TO SECOND SEND

                    The COMPARE Procedure
           Comparison of WORK.FIRST with WORK.SECOND
                       (Method=EXACT)

                      Data Set Summary

   Dataset              Created         Modified   NVar    NObs

   WORK.FIRST    25JAN04:17:23:54  25JAN04:17:23:54    35      30
   WORK.SECOND   25JAN04:17:23:54  25JAN04:17:23:54    35      28


                      Variables Summary

           Number of Variables in Common: 35.
           Number of ID Variables: 1.

                 Comparison Results for Observations

 Observation 6 in WORK.FIRST not found in WORK.SECOND:NAME=LEAD_ABL.

 Observation 10 in WORK.FIRST not found in WORK.SECOND:NAME=PHY_COM.


                      Observation Summary

            Observation     Base  Compare  ID

            First Obs          1        1  NAME=CONDUCT
            First Unequal     30       28  NAME=VISITDAY
            Last  Unequal     30       28  NAME=VISITDAY
            Last  Obs         30       28  NAME=VISITDAY
```

(continued)

```
Number of Observations in Common: 28.
Number of Observations in WORK.FIRST but not in WORK.SECOND: 2.
   Total Number of Observations Read from WORK.FIRST: 30.
   Total Number of Observations Read from WORK.SECOND: 28.

   Number of Observations with Some Compared Variables Unequal: 1.
   Number of Observations with All Compared Variables Equal: 27.

                    Values Comparison Summary

   Number of Variables Compared with All Observations Equal: 32.
   Number of Variables Compared with Some Observations Unequal: 2.
   Total Number of Values which Compare Unequal: 2.
   Maximum Difference: 1.
```

Output 5.6

```
                 Variables with Unequal Attributes

      Variable  Type  Len   Label          Ndif   MaxDif

      JUST      CHAR   10   Justification    1     1.000
      JUST      NUM     8   Justification    1     1.000
```

Output 5.7

```
               Value Comparison Results for Variables

                       ||  Variable Type
                       ||    Base     Compare
          NAME         ||    TYPE      TYPE      Diff.     % Diff
          _____  ||  _____  _____  _____  _____
                       ||
          VISITDAY     ||   1.0000    2.0000    1.0000   100.0000


                       ||  Justification
                       ||    Base     Compare
          NAME         ||    JUST      JUST      Diff.     % Diff
          _____  ||  _____  _____  _____  _____
                       ||
          VISITDAY     ||   1.0000         0   -1.0000  -100.0000
```

Output 5.5 demonstrates one key area of the output from PROC COMPARE, the comparison results for observations. This section details any observations, which in this case represent variables in the ECG data set, that occur in only one of the two data sets being compared. The programmer needs to confirm that the two observations in the original data that are no longer included in the current data set were meant to be dropped.

Output 5.6 lists the variables in the data sets being compared that have different attributes—including type, length, format, and label. In this example, the output indicates that at least one variable changed from character to numeric—definitely an issue to consider when programming against this data. Again, the programmer needs to confirm that this change in data type was intentional.

Output 5.7 details the actual differences in values. It is important when performing a PROC COMPARE that the ID statement be used. The ID statement should include all variables that identify a unique record so that it is easy to tell which records do not match. It's much easier to track down the discrepancies when you know exactly what records to look for. In this case, the variable VISITDAY changed from numeric to character (type 1 is numeric, 2 is character). It is easy to miss subtle differences in PROC CONTENTS output when checking manually. Luckily, PROC COMPARE can perform the data structure comparison simply and thoroughly.

5.8 Conclusion

Although SAS makes the import or export of data from a variety of file formats easy, there is still a human component needed to make sure that the process went as planned. Simply having a clean log that shows SAS thinks the processing went well doesn't always mean that it really did. In the end, there is no substitute for looking at the data and ensuring that the final product from your program is what was intended.

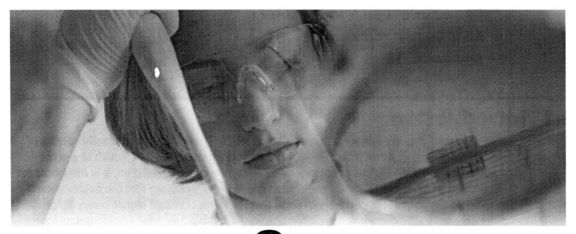

C h a p t e r **6**

Common Data Types

6.1 Introduction

Many types of data are common across clinical trials. These data types usually consist of subject characteristics and indications of the subject's general state of health at a given time. When you are validating programs that reference clinical trial data, it is important to understand what makes sense for each data type in order to ensure that the methods used to validate the program are appropriate and that the output created makes sense. Even the most detailed specifications are no substitute for understanding what potential data issues to look out for and how data interrelates. This is the knowledge that employers are looking for when asking for pharmaceutical experience. They know that an in-depth understanding of the data is the critical element to effective programming and validation in the pharmaceutical industry.

In the process of creating analyses and summary reports in support of a Clinical Study Report (CSR), analysis data sets are often created first to facilitate the creation of those reports. After those analysis data sets are created, the data is often manipulated further and summary statistics are generated in the process of creating the final tables/listings/figures (TLF) output. Throughout all of these tasks, the data needs to be considered in both the programming and validation processes. Different types of data are expected to have different structures, and the content is expected to behave in different ways. Regardless of whether you are manipulating data to create a permanently stored analysis data set or just to create a report, it is important to understand the data so you can validate the result accurately and completely. In this chapter we look at the most common data types found in clinical trials and the issues to be aware of when validating programs that reference them.

6.2 Study Populations

As discussed in Chapter 4, clinical trial data is analyzed using several different populations. Above and beyond the population of people being studied in the trial itself (subjects with a certain disease, subjects within a specific age range, etc.), studies often classify subjects into populations based on particular information collected during the clinical trial. Determining which population each subject belongs to often involves examining several types of data. Enrollment information, subject characteristics, and study drug exposure might all need to be included to determine each subject's qualification for a single population group. Because the variables that indicate each population (usually referred to as population flags) are used to determine the records that will be included in each report and analysis, it is critical that the values in these variables are correct. If these population flags are incorrect, all summary TLFs that are generated will be incorrect, even if the output is valid based on the data being used. The interpretation of those results will also be adversely affected if based on incorrect populations.

Multiple populations are often defined for a study, and there is typically one variable per population that identifies inclusion or exclusion in the population. The critical thing to remember about populations is that once a subject is part of one, that subject is always part of it. A subject should not qualify for a population in the demography data set, but not in the vital signs data set. For this reason, these flags are usually created and stored in a permanent data set so that they need to be defined and validated only once.

6.2.1 Safety

The safety population is usually defined as the group of subjects in the trial who have received at least one study treatment (dose of the study medication or device application). The validation of this data is more extensive than for any of the other populations. Since many more data points are analyzed in the safety data, it is important to be sure that all of this data is represented correctly. When checking whether a subject received study medication, you must understand all of the places in the database where receipt of study medication could be indicated. In trials where more than one study medication is given (Drug A, Drug B, and a placebo), it is important to know whether receipt of the placebo qualifies as receiving study medication. In addition, if the administration of Drug A is captured in one data set and administration of Drug B is captured in another, it is critical to check *both* data sets to determine whether or not the study drug was administered. In some cases, you need to understand what actually qualifies as having received study medication. For example, there might be two questions on the CRF: "Did the subject receive Drug A?" and "If yes, how much was taken?" Answering "yes" to the first question might not be enough to qualify as having actually received Drug A; the answer to how much was taken might need to be greater than 0. These are the kinds of details that, if not in the specification documentation, need to be questioned when validating the safety population flag.

6.2.2 Intent-to-Treat

Often the Intent-to-Treat (ITT) population includes any subject who agreed to participate in the trial (by signing an informed consent form) and who was officially included in the trial (usually by being assigned a random study ID). In many cases, these subjects are not required to have taken study medication. However, in some types of trials, this population is used to differentiate subjects who received *any* study medication (safety population) from those who received the *intended* study medication (ITT population). It is critical with this population to make sure you understand the specifications for each trial and not assume that the definition is "the same as usual." Validating this population flag could be as simple as checking to see whether a subject was assigned an official study ID, or as complicated as comparing the subject's assigned treatment group to what the dosing data indicates the subject actually received.

6.2.3 Efficacy

Efficacy population flags are often the most difficult to program and validate. They often start as a subset of another population and then include additional criteria related to the collection of efficacy data (for example, safety-evaluable subjects who also have a baseline efficacy evaluation). When these populations are created, it is often equally important to record why a subject did *not* qualify for this population. Be sure to check all specifications (including TLF mocks) to determine whether the reason for exclusion from this population is needed. If so, be sure to check what to do if multiple reasons exist. Do all reasons need to be reported or is there a hierarchy used to determine which one is reported? Consider the following example: the efficacy population is defined as safety-evaluable subjects who have a baseline efficacy evaluation within two weeks of the first dose of study medication and at least one post-dose evaluation. One safety-evaluable subject had a baseline evaluation three weeks before the first dose (so would not qualify) and had no post-dose evaluation (also would not qualify). When listing the reason this subject did not qualify for the efficacy population, you would need to know whether only one (and which one) or both reasons should be reported. Again, to effectively validate this population flag, it is critical to understand the data you are working with, all of the specifications, and how the data fits into those specifications. It is important to bring any cases where the data and the specifications do not match *exactly* to the attention of the author of the specification (usually a statistician) for clarification.

6.3 Common Data Domains

Several types of data (data domains) are common to almost all studies, regardless of differences in study designs or products being studied. It is critical to understand these data domains and how they interrelate to enable effective validation of any output created with this data. Knowing what these domains generally contain and what types of data manipulations are typically done with each facilitates validation, because you know what issues to look for.

6.3.1 Subject Demographics

The demographics data set is probably the most important data set to create correctly. Data from this data set is usually merged with all of the other data in the database before generating the reports and analyses. The main reason for this merging is to add age, sex and race to each data set that is submitted to regulatory authorities. While CDISC is often the basis for the general structure of analysis data sets containing demographics, at this time there is no absolute standard for what variables are included in the demography data set. However, there are several that are very commonly included with this data set. In general, demography data includes date of birth, sex, race and ethnicity directly from the CRF database. Age is usually calculated, although it can be captured on the CRF. In most studies, population flags are also kept with the demography data. Additionally, the analysis data sets might also add items from other data sets, such as baseline height and weight from the vital signs data set or treatment group assignment from the randomization data set.

For the data captured directly from the CRF (such as sex, race, and ethnicity), data can be either text or codes (for example, "1" represents Male and "2" represents Female). In cases where coded values are decoded, it is critical to validate the decoded values. Using PROC FREQ to create a crosstabulation of the coded value versus the decoded value does that efficiently (see Chapter 4 for an example). To validate age calculations, it is not enough simply to check a few of the numbers manually. You need to understand the inclusion criteria for the trial as well. If the inclusion criteria state that subjects should be 18 to 59 years old, you should not see any 3-year-olds in the data. Similar checks for reasonable data values should be considered when validating any demographic variable.

6.3.2 Inclusion/Exclusion Criteria

The data for this domain can vary depending on the design of the CRF. In some cases, this data simply includes a question regarding whether all of the inclusion and exclusion criteria were met, and if not, which criteria are exceptions. In other cases, this data includes yes/no checks for each individual inclusion and exclusion criterion. With the advent of CDISC, the only required data submitted for this domain consists of exceptions to the inclusion and exclusion criteria.

In cases where each criterion is captured, you might need to cross-check some of the criteria to other data in the database. For example, a subject's age needs to be verified as meeting the criteria, even if the check box value for that criterion is "yes." In addition, if waiver information is captured in a separate data set and one of the inclusion or exclusion criteria is not met, you probably need to ensure that there is waiver information directly associated with the unmet criterion. In general, the responses to all inclusion criteria should be "yes" and the responses to all exclusion criteria should be "no." However, there are some cases where the questions might be phrased in the reverse so that the opposite is true. You need to review the CRF and understand each question to ensure that you validate your results correctly.

6.3.3 Subject Disposition

Subject disposition is usually thought of as the reason that a subject discontinued or stopped participating in the clinical trial. Did the subject take the study drug for the full term of the trial? If not, why? Although this is the main topic in the disposition domain, it is not the only information included in study disposition. In some studies where a subject completes a treatment period and then is followed for additional information after treatment is finished, there might be more than one study discontinuation status. There is often one status when a subject completes the dosing portion of the trial, and then a separate status when the subject completes the follow-up period. In addition to discontinuation status, CDISC also considers informed consent status and randomization status to fall within this data domain. With each of these disposition categories, the date at which these events took place is also collected. The two items to pay particular attention to when working with and validating this data are the informed consent status and the dates relative to the first dose of study treatment.

It is critical to understand the overall status of the trial, particularly when you are dealing with reasons for study discontinuation. If one of the reasons that a subject discontinued is reported as "completed three-year follow-up," you need to know whether that response is even possible. If the study started enrolling subjects only two years ago, this would be an impossible response. There might be similar issues when you look at randomization status. If the study you are working with also collects the reason that a subject is not randomized, you might need to make sure that those reasons also make sense compared to other data in the database. For example, if the reason the subject is not randomized is reported as "inclusion criteria not met," you might need to cross-check against the inclusion data to make sure this is the case.

The other critical aspect of disposition data that needs to be checked for reasonable values is the date of the event (inclusion, randomization, or discontinuation) relative to the date that the first study treatment was administered. While subtracting the event date from the first treatment date will not create any errors in your log, part of the validation process also involves making sure the result makes sense. You should not have discontinuation dates prior to the first treatment, nor should patients be randomized into the trial after the first treatment. Cases where key dates don't make sense relative to one another should be brought to the attention of the appropriate project team members who can resolve data issues.

6.3.4 Medical History

At the onset of each subject's participation in a study, the investigator takes an inventory of any relevant medical events that the subject has experienced prior to starting the trial. This information can be captured in a variety of ways that can affect the type of validation effort needed to ensure that the data and any analyses are correct. In general, for medical history data to be summarized in tables, the data needs to be categorized in some way. The main method for this categorization is to collect the data based on body system as captured on the CRF. Although the medical history categories might change, a typical example of medical history body system categories is as follows:

- Dermatologic

- Head, eyes, ears, nose and throat (HEENT)

- Cardiovascular

- Pulmonary

- Gastrointestinal

- Hepatic / Renal

- Genitourinary / Gynecological

- CNS

- Hematologic / Oncologic

- Metabolic / Endocrine

- Allergies

These body systems can be reported in the database either as full text representations of each system or as a body system code (for example, "1" represents Dermatologic). If you need to decode the body systems, it is important to verify that these decoded categories are correct. In most cases where categories are preprinted on the CRF, there is also a question such as "any events reported?" If the answer to this kind of question is "yes," then there should also be a specific finding listed. If summary tables report cases where this variable is "yes," then it is important that the variable be accurate. When validating, you need to ensure that this status variable is "yes" in every case where a finding is specified, and that the status is "no" where there is no finding.

The other method for categorizing medical history events is to code the event descriptions using an electronic event dictionary such as the Medical Dictionary for Regulated Activities (MedDRA). These dictionaries allow knowledgeable professionals to match verbatim text responses to consistent terms for accurate categorization and reporting. If a dictionary is used to code medical history events, it is important to ensure that every event listed has been coded.

In addition to ensuring that all events have body systems or dictionary terms associated with them, you might also be required to impute partially missing dates. Often subjects know what month and year an event happened, but they might not remember the exact day. For this reason, dates are usually captured in character variables so that partial dates can be reported. However, if you are required to calculate how long ago a given event happened, you need a complete, numeric date for the calculation. It is important to have and understand any rules for imputing missing date parts before imputing dates and then validating the results. Usually the most conservative rules are applied, which involve assuming the event started as far from the first treatment as possible (so if the day of the month is missing, you would use the first of the month to impute a complete, numeric date). If stop dates are also imputed, it is critical to check that any imputed dates still make sense when compared to the study schedule. If an imputed end date ends up *after* the first dose of the study treatment, it might indicate a problem with the imputation rule. If both the start and end dates are imputed, it is important to ensure that the start date is still before the end date. In addition to actually imputing the dates, it is important to flag any dates that are imputed so you can differentiate actual dates from imputed dates. Once again, validation is not just a matter of making sure your SAS logs are free from errors and warnings, but making sure that the result makes sense.

6.3.5 Physical Examination

Physical examination data is very similar to medical history data in that the investigator takes an inventory of any relevant medical events that the subject is experiencing. The major difference is in the timing. Medical history records events that happened before the start of the clinical trial, whereas physical exams record events occurring during or immediately before the clinical trial. If the body system categories are preprinted on the page, they might be slightly different from those listed on the medical history page. They are often a bit more specific (for example, Chest and Heart might be listed rather than just Cardiovascular).

In addition, physical exams are often done several times over the course of a trial rather than just once at the beginning. Depending on what data is collected, you might need to check data across visits. You need to understand how the exam data is recorded and how data from each visit might relate to similar data at other visits. For example, if information about each body system is collected across three visits, and there are findings at visit one, should you expect to have findings for the same body system across the other two visits? In addition, you might need to check that the visits happened when they were scheduled to be done. If an exam was supposed to be completed one day after dosing, is it a problem if it happened three days after dosing?

6.3.6 Vital Signs

Information regarding a subject's vital signs (usually including heart rate, blood pressure, respiration rate, temperature, height, and weight) is usually collected multiple times over the course of a clinical trial. Minimally, this data is collected once before study treatment is administered and once after. In longer, more complex trials, vital signs are usually collected more often (for example, once per visit). Regardless of how many times vital signs are collected, one key timepoint that needs to be established is baseline. In general, the baseline values are those prior to study treatment. More specifically, baseline can be defined as either the last non-missing value before study treatment or the values reported at a baseline visit. If more than one set of vital sign values is collected prior to the first study treatment, there might be more specific rules for determining baseline values. For example, if vital signs were collected at a screening visit and a baseline visit, and the respiration rate was collected at screening but not at baseline, should the screening respiration value be used as the baseline value? These are the detailed rules that you need to understand in order to effectively validate output based on vital signs data.

After baseline values have been established, change from baseline is often calculated at subsequent post-treatment timepoints. When validating these values, it is important to understand what values make sense for each parameter. Does a 30-point increase in heart rate seem reasonable when you consider that the drug being studied is supposed to reduce anxiety? However, if you were to see the same data in a study for a drug that is used to revive patients after anesthesia, your conclusion might be different. Using PROC FREQ to see the range of values for each parameter will help you pick out values that look suspicious for the data you are working with.

Another area that needs to be validated is the conversion of results from one unit to another. Temperature might be reported in both Celsius and Fahrenheit; weight might be reported in both pounds and kilograms. To analyze this data effectively, all data must be in the same units. Again, it is not enough that the logic follows specification and there are no errors in the log. After all data has been converted to a single unit, it is critical to look at that data (again PROC FREQ works well for this) and make sure that the values are reasonable. Often the wrong unit is recorded in the database, and when the values are reviewed in total, it is obvious where the data needs to be corrected. Data that includes a 175 kilogram subject would be reasonable only if the study were looking at a treatment for obesity.

Another important aspect of working with vital sign data is the concept of normal ranges and flagging data that falls outside of these ranges. Normal ranges describe the values considered normal for each parameter, and values that fall outside of these ranges are considered either low or high. For example, heart rate might be considered normal between 50 and 120 beats per minute. Any value below 50 would be considered low, whereas any value above 120 would be considered high. Generating crosstabulations with PROC FREQ to compare the flag value to the actual value is a good way to ensure that the flags are assigned correctly. In addition, it might be helpful to print any values that are out of range to ensure that they are not so far out of range as to be impossible (a heart rate of 5 beats per minute is likely a data issue).

When you deal with data that is collected across multiple visits, it is often important to know when the data was collected relative to when study treatment was administered. If vital signs were supposed to be collected one hour before treatment and one hour after, it might be important to confirm that the second measurement really was taken after treatment. It might also be important to check that visits happened when they were supposed to. For example, if data was supposed to be collected on study days one and five, and the data was actually collected on days one and ten, is the data that was collected on day ten still valid for analysis?

6.3.7 Treatment Exposure

Exposure to study treatment is one of the most important areas of information in a clinical trial. Many aspects of this information make it critical for you to understand the design of the trial and all specifications. It is not enough to simply follow specifications in order to program and validate code that uses this data. If you do not understand the study design and data expectations, you will not be able to produce accurate output. Knowing how much study medication a subject is supposed to receive and at what timepoints is critical in making sure that the data makes sense.

In many cases, treatment must be given at specific intervals, and the margin for deviation from that interval varies. Similar to checking vital sign data timepoints, you might need to make sure that treatments were administered as scheduled in the study protocol. If timepoints are close together (the drug is administered every hour for six hours), the margin for deviation might be as small as five minutes. In contrast, if treatments are administered once per month, deviations of six days might be permissible. By understanding the dosing schedule and then looking at the data itself, you can determine whether the data for any subjects does not meet the expectations in the programming specifications. If data does not meet the specifications, a statistician might need to provide input on how to deal with it appropriately. It is important to make note of any issues with subjects or timepoints so you can make sure this data is handled appropriately in other programs that make assumptions about how subjects are dosed.

In other cases, the treatment interval is less important than the amount of treatment actually received. Determining the treatment actually received might be as simple as adding the number of pills taken or volume of liquid injected, or it might involve more complex calculations. Actual dose received might be a function of how many milligrams of drug were ingested versus a subject's weight, body mass index, or body surface area. In these more complicated calculations, it is necessary to make sure that the components of the calculation make sense and that the calculation itself was performed correctly. It is important to understand what a reasonable subject weight is, what the scheduled dose in milligrams is, and what the expected actual dose should be so that you can make sure the results of your actual dose calculation are accurate.

In randomized trials, you might also need to determine whether the subject actually received the treatment that was assigned. If a subject was supposed to get Drug A but received Drug B instead, there are likely to be implications for how the data for that subject gets analyzed throughout the study. It is important to identify any problem subjects like this to make sure that their data is handled correctly in *all* programs (not just those related specifically to reporting treatment information).

6.3.8 Concomitant Medications

Concomitant, or concurrent, medications are any medications other than the study treatment taken by the subject during the course of the study. The names of the medications themselves are usually collected as verbatim text fields that are coded using an electronic dictionary such as the World Health Organization Drug Reference List (WHODRL) to classify medications by therapeutic class and preferred term. It is critical for all data to be coded before reporting. In addition to the name of the drug, the date the subject started the medication as well as the date he or she stopped are usually recorded. Other information, such as the reason for the medication (or indication), route of administration, dose, and frequency, might be recorded. This information can either be verbatim text or prespecified on the CRF. If this data is collected in the database as a code (e.g., for route of administration, 1 = "oral," 2 = "injection," 3 = "topical," etc.), it is critical to make sure that the values are decoded correctly.

Start and stop dates for medications are often partially or completely missing. Medications that subjects started five years ago might only have a month and year present ("JAN2002") and medications that the subject is still taking when the clinical trial completes might have no end date reported at all. These partial dates often have the missing parts imputed so that they can be made into a numeric date and date math can be performed. As with other types of data where partial dates are imputed, it is important to make sure that the resulting dates make sense. A missing month and day should not be imputed to a full date that does not make sense with the study timeline. In addition, medication start and stop dates should not be imputed such that the start date occurs after the stop date.

After valid numeric start and stop dates are available for each medication, the relative study day for start and stop, as well as the duration of the medication, are usually calculated. Typically, medications are also categorized by when they were taken during the trial. Medications started before the study treatment would be categorized as "prior," medications started during the study period would be categorized as "during," and medications started within thirty days after the last study treatment would be categorized as "post." After you have the relative study day of the start of the medication, it is fairly easy to categorize the start as prior, during or post. It is important to check that these two variables correspond to one another (prior medications should have a negative study start day, during and post medications should have positive days). Medications that started more than thirty days after the last study treatment might not need to be included in any analyses. It is important to check these details in the specifications before attempting to validate this data.

6.3.9 Adverse Events

Except for treatment exposure, adverse event data frequently gets the most focus in clinical trials. This data is the primary indication of how safe the study treatment is. While there are some variations in how adverse event data is collected, the key information that is almost always collected is as follows:

- Description of the event—usually as a verbatim text field

- Event start date—start time as well, if appropriate

- Event end date—end time, if appropriate, as well as an indication of whether the event was ongoing at the end of the trial

- Severity—usually "mild," "moderate," or "severe"; for cancer trials usually also includes the National Cancer Institute (NCI) Common Toxicity Criteria (CTC)

- Seriousness—a "yes" or "no" field that should not be confused with severity

- Relation to study treatment—usually "not related," "possibly related," "definitely related," or "unknown"

- Action taken—often indicates what action was taken with study treatment (treatment was delayed, stopped, or not changed)

- Outcome—usually "resolved," "resolved with sequelae," "unresolved," or "fatal"

It is critical to understand how these pieces of information interrelate both with each other within the adverse events data set as well as with other data in the trial. While data points such as relation to study treatment might need only a simple check to make sure that valid values are reported, others need much more careful review. Starting with the event description, the following discussion covers the more complex data points and the critical elements of each.

As with concomitant medications and medical history, the description of the adverse event must be matched with a common term ("coded") using an electronic dictionary such as MedDRA to allow for summarization and reporting. Also similar to these other data sets, the event start and stop day relative to the first dose of study treatment are often calculated. To do these date calculations, the event dates need to be complete numeric dates. The imputation rules for these dates are often more complex than those used for dates such as medical history event start, because it is much more important for the adverse event dates to fit logically within the clinical trial timeline. In these cases, it is important to find records in the data that qualify for each step in the logic and manually review the outcome to make sure it makes sense. For example, the rule for imputing a missing event start day when the month and year are present might be as follows:

- If the month and year are the same as the year and month of the first day on treatment, then the start date of treatment is assigned to the missing day.

- If the month and year are before the year and month of the first day on treatment, then the last day of the month is assigned to the missing day.

- If the month and year are after the year and month of the first day on treatment, then the first day of the month is assigned to the missing day.

In this case, you should search the data set for data where the start date is missing only the day, and then find one of each where the month and year are before, the same, and after the first day of study treatment. After you have imputed the dates to be complete dates, you should review the results to make sure that the day of the month was assigned as the specification dictates. In all cases you need to make sure that the end date is after the start date. These dates can sometimes be transposed when events occur around the end of the year (start in December and end in January) because the year is often recorded incorrectly.

The severity of an event indicates how intense the event is. It is important to understand how this data is collected, as it varies based on the indication being studied in the clinical trial. In most trials not related to cancer, this data is typically as simple as "mild," "moderate," or "severe." However, in cancer trials, CTC grades that range from zero (normal) to five (fatal) are often reported either in place of or in addition to the simpler severity classifications. In these cases, it is important to have a general understanding of the range in grades so you know not to expect a Grade 0 adverse event. In addition, if you see a Grade 5 event, you should also expect that the outcome of the event would be listed as "fatal."

While seemingly similar to severity, seriousness is a separate measure of the overall magnitude of the adverse event. It is important to understand that the definition of "serious" for adverse events includes any event that is life-threatening or results in hospitalization, birth defects, or death. It is possible to have a "severe" headache that is not serious. By the same token, it is possible to have "moderate" chest pain that results in hospitalization and is therefore considered "serious." By understanding the definition of seriousness, you can better evaluate the quality of the data and subsequently validate your code. For example, any cases where the event outcome is "fatal" should be considered as "severe." Besides the adverse event data, you might also need to cross-check the disposition data (the reason for discontinuation of study treatment would likely be "death") and any information collected on a separate CRF page related to death. Programmers are expected to know that they must make these kinds of checks, so this type of information will not necessarily be detailed in the specifications. If you don't check that the data you are working with is consistent, recipients of your output might assume that the code generating that output is incorrect.

Action taken with study medication is another data point within adverse events data that might need to be cross-checked with data from other domains. For example, if the action taken indicates that study treatment was stopped, you might need to check that no treatment was administered after the end date of the event. Similarly, the reason for study treatment discontinuation might need to be listed as "adverse event." When you are programming analysis data sets, these cross-domain inconsistencies might not be apparent. However, when an adverse event summary table indicates that ten subjects discontinued treatment due to an adverse event, but the subject disposition table shows only nine subjects discontinued due to adverse events, the validity of the tables might be questioned. By checking that related data is consistent early in the process, you can address these questions before they become an issue.

Finally, the outcome of the adverse event needs to be checked for consistency with other data points within the adverse events domain, as well as with other data domains in the study. For example, if the outcome is "resolved," then there should be an end date reported for the event. Similarly, if the outcome is "unresolved," then the end date should be blank. All data points that have the potential to indicate that the event was "fatal" (severity and seriousness) should align, as well as data from other data domains as discussed earlier. Again, by making sure that related data is consistent, you avoid reporting discrepancies that will cause the quality of the reports to come into question.

6.3.10 Clinical Laboratory Data

Perhaps the most challenging data collected in a clinical trial is the laboratory data collected for safety review (usually including blood and urine analysis). Although other types of data can also be complex to work with, lab data has the extra component of volume. For each timepoint where data is collected, the results of the blood analysis are broken into major types (hematology and chemistry), and within each of those, multiple tests can be analyzed. Typical hematology data includes tests on such things as hemoglobin, hematocrit, platelets, red blood cells (RBC), white blood cells (WBC) and each of the WBC components (neutrophils, basophils, eosinophils, lymphocytes, and monocytes). Chemistry data often includes tests for such things as sodium, glucose, potassium, calcium, albumin, creatinine, bilirubin, alkaline phosphatase, and others. When hematology and chemistry data are collected in the same data set, it is not hard to see why it is often the largest data set in the database.

Lab data can be collected for a clinical trial in two ways: on the CRF or through a centralized laboratory. When collected on the CRF, the blood and/or urine samples are usually sent to a local laboratory (often within the clinic or hospital where the subject is receiving study treatment) and the results are recorded directly on the CRF page. An abbreviated example of a CRF page is shown in Example 6.1.

Example 6.1

CLINICAL LABORATORY ASSESSMENTS								
(Within 3 Days Prior to Study Drug Administration on Day 1)								

Please record the name of the laboratory that was used: _____

Date of Collection: __ __ __ __ __ __ __ __ __   Time of Collection: __ __ : __ __
          d d m m m y y y y   (24-Hour Clock)

Serum Chemistry	Unit	Lab Result	Check if this lab value is associated with an AE	Serum Chemistry	Unit	Lab Result	Check if this lab value is associated with an AE
Sodium	☐ mEq/L ☐ mmol/L ☐ mg/dL ☐ other: _____		☐ı	Bilirubin	☐ mg/dL ☐ umol/L ☐ g/dL ☐ other: _____		☐ı
Potassium	☐ mEq/L ☐ mmol/L ☐ other: _____		☐ı	Alkaline Phosphatase	☐ IU/L = U/L = Units/L ☐ other: _____		☐ı
Albumin	☐ g/dL ☐ g/L ☐ mg/dL ☐ other: ____		☐ı	Calcium	☐ mg/dL ☐ mmol/L ☐ mEq/L ☐ other: _____		☐ı

Alternately, samples can be sent to a centrally located laboratory to be analyzed and recorded in a database. These results are usually sent as an electronic file (separate from the main CRF database) to the group who maintains the main CRF database. In general, it is much less complicated to work with data from a central laboratory because the data is more consistent. The following discussion treats lab data in detail as if the data had been collected on the CRF, with the understanding that many of the issues that occur in CRF data do not occur in data received from a central laboratory.

As with other data collected at multiple timepoints throughout a trial, it is important to understand the study schedule. You need to know when lab samples are supposed to be collected and how critical it is for those samples to be collected on time. As discussed with vital sign data, baseline values need to be established and change from baseline needs to be calculated and checked for reasonable values. In addition, you must consider the following two key components when programming and validating lab data.

- Standard units—All results for each test must be analyzed in the same unit.

- Normal ranges—Results need to be compared to these ranges and categorized as normal, low or high.

Converting all results to standard units is perhaps one of the most challenging aspects of working with local lab data. This is one area where collecting data through a central laboratory is a huge advantage, because data from a single source uses a single set of units.

6.3.10.1 Standardizing Units

Often during the course of a clinical trial, laboratory data is collected in multiple locations. Different sites might use their own labs, or subjects from the same site might have samples taken and analyzed at different labs. Different laboratories can analyze samples in different units—either conventional units (used regularly in the United States) or Standard International (SI) units (a global standard for reporting laboratory results, usually metric). A related example of conventional versus international units is weight collected in pounds versus kilograms. Although the collection of lab results in SI units is becoming more common, it is not an absolute standard as far as analysis at the laboratory yet. In contrast, when results are filed outside of the United States, the use of SI units for reporting lab values is mandatory. As a result, most data collected using conventional units gets converted to SI units before submission. Regardless of the units being used to report the data, all results must be reported in the *same* unit for each test, or analysis would be meaningless. To enable conversion of results from one unit to another, conversion factors (the numeric multiplier or divisor applied to a value that results in a new value in the target unit) are used. These factors might be provided in documentation that needs to be applied directly in SAS code, or they might be maintained in a database. It is critical to make sure that these factors are applied correctly and that the resulting values make sense. Not only do you need to make sure that any formulas are applied as the specifications dictate, but you also need to make sure the results are not reported in the wrong unit (the result is truly "3," but the incorrect unit is associated with that value). In many cases, these errors are not noticed until all values are converted to the same unit and then these values become outliers.

There are several ways to validate the transformation of units. One way is to use PROC FREQ to cross-check each unit with values (TABLE testname*result / LIST;). Although this can be a useful tool, manually reviewing a list of that magnitude can be a daunting task. Another method to facilitate the validation of this data is to graph it so that outlying values are easy to find with a quick visual review.

Using PROC UNIVARIATE in association with several ODS statements can provide basic graphs that can be reviewed very easily by sight. Let's look at the code and the accompanying output with the following assumptions:

1. the data set containing the lab data is called LABS

2. the LABS data set is sorted by lab test using the variable LBTEST

3. the variable containing the standardized laboratory test value is called LBSTRESN

Example 6.2

```
ods select plots;
proc univariate data = LABS plots;
    by lbtest;
    var lbstresn;
    title "Check for extreme lab values";
run;
```

Output 6.1 and 6.2 contain the output from PROC UNIVARIATE. Use of the PLOT statement provides three different types of output:

1. Histogram—This graph displays all of the values from the data using the vertical axis to identify value. Note that the longer horizontal lines represent data that is similar. The longer the horizontal graphed line, the more subjects experienced results of the same value.

2. Box plot—This graph displays a condensed representation of the trend of the data. The plus represents the mean value found. The box represents the standard deviation from the mean. The whiskers above and below the box show outliers (i.e., values that are far from the mean).

3. Normal probability plot—This graph shows the normal distribution of values and any departures from normal. The center of plot (point 0) is the point at which most values occur. Prior to and past 0 are values distributed from the mean.

Output 6.1

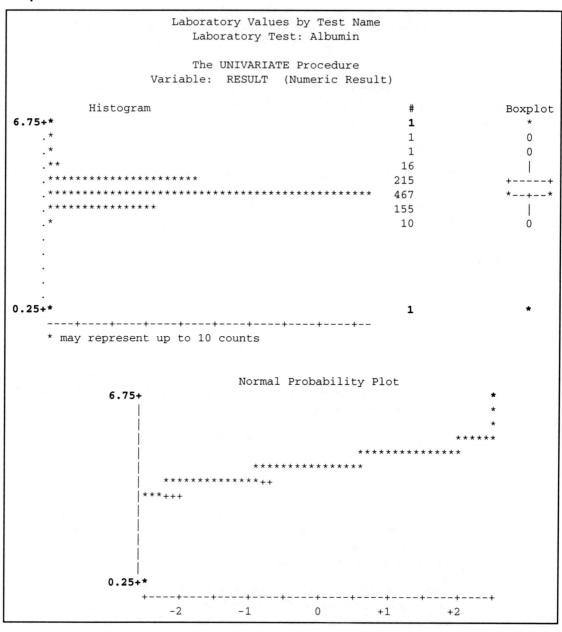

Output 6.2

```
                        Laboratory Values by Test Name
                        Laboratory Test: Serum Sodium

                           The UNIVARIATE Procedure
                        Variable:  RESULT   (Numeric Result)

              Histogram                                #        Boxplot
      181+*                                            1           *
         .
         .
         .
         .
         .
         .
         .
      159+
         .
         .*                                            1           0
         .*                                            5           0
       ***                                            15           0
        .**********                                   63           |
        .*************************                   173        +-----+
        .*************************************************     273       *--+--*
        .****************************************            242        +-----+
        .*************                                83           |
      137+**                                          12           0
         ----+----+----+----+----+----+----+----+----+-
          * may represent up to 6 counts
```

(continued)

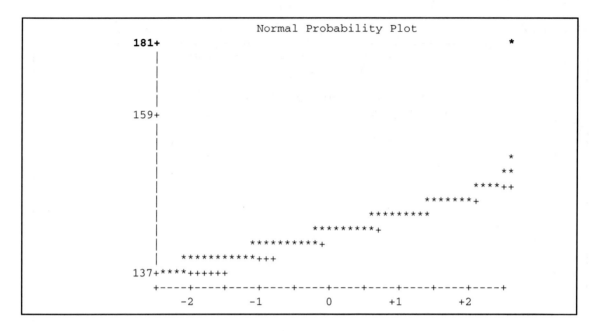

The obviously high or low values are shown in bold. Notice in Output 6.1 that the values of 6.75 and 2.5 are drastically far away from the normal distribution. These might be cases where either the unit conversions were done incorrectly or the original result was reported in the wrong unit. In either case, these values need to be investigated during the validation process. Using this method is a basic, quick way of viewing all of the data at the same time so the identification of outliers and potential data problems can be accomplished easily and effectively.

6.3.10.2 Applying Normal Ranges
Similar to vital signs data, each lab test has a range within which values are considered normal. Normal ranges for lab data are challenging, because they can differ by lab test and other factors. They might vary depending on the subject's gender or age (men between the ages of 18 and 64 might have a different normal range for albumin than women over 65). In addition, due mainly to differences in the equipment used to test the actual samples, normal ranges can vary depending on the laboratory performing the analysis. When combined with the task of ensuring that both the normal ranges and the results are in the same unit, the validation of this data takes on a whole new level of complexity.

There are several ways to validate the consistency of the results in a common unit and the addition of the normal ranges to the laboratory data. Using SAS/GRAPH software in association with several ODS statements provides more detailed graphs that can be reviewed very easily by sight. In addition, SAS/GRAPH allows for the addition of the normal ranges to the output. This makes finding the outliers that much easier. Let's look at the code and the accompanying output with the following assumptions:

- the data set containing the lab data is called LABS

- the LABS data set is sorted by lab test using the variable LBTEST

- the variable containing the laboratory test value is called LBSTRESN

```
**-------------------------------------------------------------**
**   CREATE THE PLOT                                           **;
**-------------------------------------------------------------**;
** GRAPHING OPTIONS **;
axis1 label = (angle=90 "Result")
      offset= (2);

axis2 label = ('Visit')
      order = (1 to 3 by 1)
      value = ('Visit 0' 'Visit 2' 'Visit 3')
      offset= (2);

symbol1  value=star color=black h=2.00 width=2;
symbol2  value=dot color=black h=1.50;

** SYSTEM OPTIONS **;
options nodate nonumber nobyline orientation = landscape;
goptions hsize=9.0in vsize=5.5000in;

ods listing close ;
ods escapechar='^' ;
ods rtf  file=" lab_graphs.rtf"
         nogtitle nogfootnote;

%MACRO GRAPH(test);

   data graph;
     set labs (where = (upcase(lbtest)= "&test")) end=end;

  ** SEND THE NORMAL RANGE HI AND LO VALUES TO MACRO VARIABLES **;
     if end then
       do;
          if lbstnrlo ne . then call symput("lo",put(lbstnrlo,best1 2.));
          else call symput("lo",put(0,best12.));

          if lbstnrhi ne . then call symput("hi",put(lbstnrhi,best1 2.));
          else call symput("hi",put(0,best12.));
       end;
   run;
```

```
proc gplot data = graph;
    plot lbstresn * visitnum /
    vaxis=axis1
              haxis=axis2
    noframe
    vref = &lo. &hi.
    lvref = (2 4);
quit;

%MEND GRAPH;
%graph(ALBUMIN)
%graph(SERUM SODIUM)

ods rtf close ;
ods listing ;
```

Output 6.3

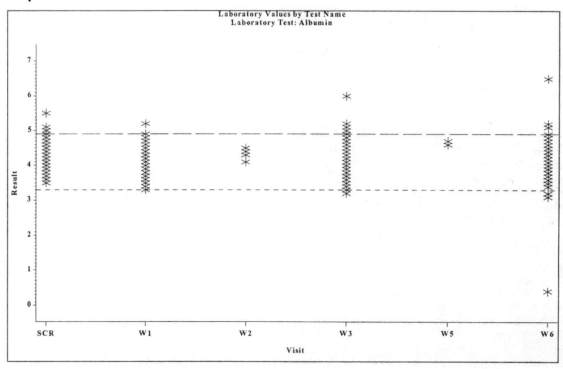

Output 6.4

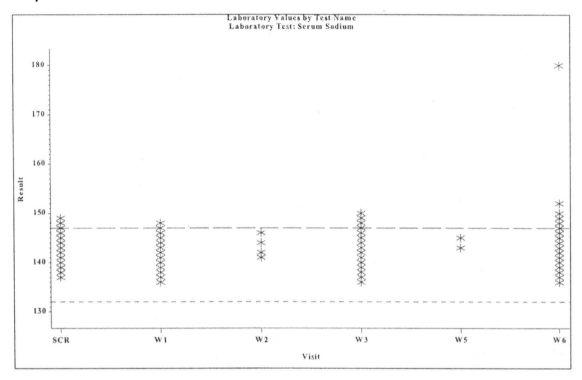

Let's break down the code step by step and then review the output:

Step 1. Setting up the axes:

The AXIS1 statement sets up the defaults for printing the results along the Y axis. The AXIS2 statement allows for three visits along the X axis and spreads them out evenly. The SYMBOL1 and SYMBOL2 statements define the characters to be used when plotting the individual values of the lab results variable LBSTRESN and VISITNUM on the graph.

Step 2. Setting system and graphing options:

The system and graphing options used for this graphing are as follows:

NODATE—removes the date from the titles

NONUMBER—removes the page number from the titles

NOBYLINE—removes the by line description from the titles

ORIENTATION=LANDSCAPE—flips the orientation of the graph to a landscape presentation

HSIZE—displays the horizontal axis using 9 inches

VSIZE—displays the vertical axis using 5.5 inches

Step 3. ODS statements:

The ODS statements used to produce the graphs are typical ODS statements. They redirect the output from the SAS .LST file to an RTF file with a name of your choosing. The important elements to notice in the ODS RTF statement are the use of the options NOGTITLE and NOGFOOTNOTE. Without these two options, SAS includes all of the TITLE and FOOTNOTE statements in the "picture" that it creates in the RTF file. With the options turned off, all TITLE and FOOTNOTE statements appear as titles and footnotes in the header and footer sections of the output, leaving only the graph as the "picture" in the RTF file. This allows for consistency and continuity of all of the output, which is particularly important when your output file type is RTF (these graphs can be included in other Word documents).

Step 4. Preparing the data:

The DATA step at the beginning of the macro performs several tasks. First, a new data set is created that is subsetted to the laboratory test being passed into the macro. Second, the low and high ranges of normal are set into macro variables. These values are used in the graphing step to set reference lines on the graphs for the LOW and HIGH values. Note that if normal ranges differ across records in the data set, only the last one will be used for the purposes of this graph. Since this graph will be used primarily as a validation tool, this representation should be close enough for the purposes of identifying gross outliers and general consistency.

Step 5. Graphing the values:

The PROC GPLOT statement begins the graphing of the values, by lab test, for each record and visit.

The following are important elements of the PLOT statement:

VREF =&lo. &hi.   These are the vertical axis reference lines that are to be graphed on the plot. These values resolve to the LOW and HIGH normal values captured in the macro variables.

LVREF (2 4)   This statement tells SAS to use different line types for each of the normal ranges.

Output 6.3 and 6.4 display the output from PROC GPLOT. Each column of the output represents a visit at which the laboratory values were collected. Notice that there are two reference lines on each graph. The short dotted line represents the low value within the normal range, whereas the longer dotted line is the high value within the normal range. After all of the values found in the data are plotted, it is very easy to determine the values outside the normal range. Notice in Output 6.4 that the highest value is well above 30 points from the norm. In this case, the test for sodium is one of the tests where values that stray far from the normal range rapidly become impossible for living people. In this particular case, sodium values much above 150 can be life-threatening or physiologically impossible. These graphs, as with the previous PROC UNIVARIATE, are very helpful in finding data issues and validating data quickly and effectively.

The preceding example, in addition to helping with validation for the normal ranges, can be applied to the standardization of the values and units. By simply changing the graphing to plot the conventional units and the new standardized units, you can efficiently review the conversion by reviewing the output side by side. If the conversion was done correctly, the graphs will appear to display the same trends.

6.4 Conclusion

As we've seen in this chapter, there are many types of data collected in clinical trials, and understanding each one is critical to the validation process. By understanding the trial design as well as how the information being collected is expected to be reported, you can effectively check that both the data and the code that manipulates that data are correct. Clinical programmers are expected to look beyond the explicit specifications to understand what makes sense in both the data and the results. Whereas this chapter discussed key items to look for when validating specific types of data, the next chapter discusses how to validate the final results generated from that data.

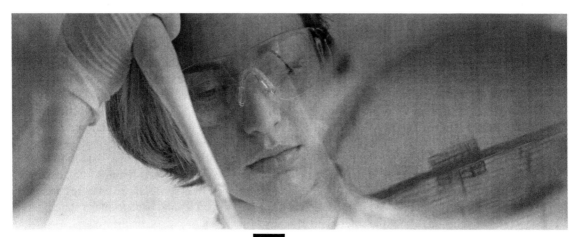

Chapter 7

Reporting and Statistics

7.1 Introduction

For all of the seeming variation in the data collected and the methods of collection in clinical trials, the reports generated on much of this data are surprisingly similar. Reports on subject demographics, relevant medical history, physical exam findings, laboratory test results, and much other information are usually generated using the same summary statistics. In many cases, the programming involves reporting the summary statistics from PROC FREQ or PROC MEANS (PROC UNIVARIATE), or both. The techniques for summarizing the data and putting it together for the report are the same regardless of the output file type (text files, RTF, PDF, etc.) or layout (portrait or landscape, data in rows vs. columns, etc.). The validation of these summary reports and data listings often constitutes the bulk of the validation effort done for a project. In essence, these analyses are the final product that is added to the Clinical Trial Report (CTR) and used to make statements and conclusions about the safety and efficacy of the drug or device being studied.

As mentioned in Chapter 2, there are generally two approaches to validation—independent programming and peer review. Before either of these approaches comes into play, the programmer who is responsible for generating the final production output must validate his or her own work. Regardless of the data being analyzed or reported, and regardless of whether you are responsible for the production output or for validating someone else's output, there are general principals that apply to validating different categories of output, such as tables, listings, or figures.

7.2 Pre-Output Validation Steps

One of the key elements of the validation process is the review of SAS code and SAS logs. No matter what type of output you are creating or the data with which you create it, the code itself needs to make sense and the log needs to be free of errors and warnings. Although the final output is the ultimate product being validated, starting validation with the code and the log increases the probability that the final product will be accurate and correct.

7.2.1 Code Review

As mentioned in Chapter 3, it is critical that code be easy to read and contain enough comments to allow easy understanding of what is being done (and sometimes why). It is good practice to review your own code after it is written to make sure that the comments make sense and are sufficient to explain what is being done. Regardless of whether you are reviewing your own code or your peer's as part of the validation process, code review (reviewing the .SAS file) is an important step, and the final code should meet the following criteria:

1. Is the code readable and understandable?

2. Are there sufficient comments such that another programmer could read and understand what is happening?

3. Is there a logical and reasonable flow to the program?

4. Does the code make sense in relation to the specifications? Is it reasonable to assume that the final outcome being created from this code would be accurate?

5. Are there any flaws or weaknesses in logic where the code could fail?

6. Does the code adhere to the company standards?

It is important that the code be reviewed with these questions in mind. If the code itself is able to pass these criteria favorably, you are less likely to have major issues with the final output, and any minor issues will be much easier to trace.

7.2.2 Log Review

Log review is another important step in the validation process. Any messages of concern can be cause for speculation about the accuracy of the final output. Every SAS log should be scanned and reviewed for SAS notes, warnings, and errors. You might want to consider looking for, at the very least, messages that start with the following keywords:

ERROR

WARNING

INFO: Character

INFO: The variable

NOTE: At least

NOTE: Character

NOTE: Division

NOTE: Mathematical

NOTE: Merge

NOTE: Missing

NOTE: NOSPOOL

NOTE: Numeric

NOTE: Variable

Although the warning and error messages are clear problems, the notes listed above are often more subtle indications that the data or the code is not behaving as expected. Although SAS is able to continue processing the data, it might not be doing what you really intended. It is critical to understand what each of these notes means and to ensure that the results are what was intended. Even if SAS handles the data correctly, it is best that you adjust your code so that these notes do not appear. By doing so, you prevent the notes from being a cause for concern if code needs to be run in the future.

In addition to simply checking for notes and warnings, it is important to follow the number of observations from one step to another. It is possible to receive unexpected final results due to issues in the data or unexpected problems with the code logic, even though the code executes with no notes or warnings. In many cases such problems are revealed by the number of observations being different than expected. Before you review the final output, it is critical to review the log to make sure the number of observations flowing into and out of each data step or procedure makes logical sense. Chances are that if the number of observations doesn't make sense, the final output won't make sense either.

7.3 Output Validation Steps

Across different types of output and different types of data, similar processes are used for the validation of the final output. Although some steps might differ in the way they are completed for different types of output being reviewed, it is still important to complete each step. The following sections explain what validation steps need to occur and, in general, how to go about completing them.

7.3.1 Understanding the Data

Before you validate any kind of output, it is critical that you first have a good understanding of the data being used to create that output. A program can run without errors and generate a pretty summary table, but if the data being presented do not make sense, the validation process can stop right there. For example, sex can be reported as male or female, but if the current study is about a birth control product for teenage girls, it would not make sense to see males in the demographic summary table.

Although creating the analysis data set often gives you a very good understanding of the data, that process does not often reveal trends in the data the way creating summary statistics can. In addition, you might be responsible for creating summary reports with data you have not worked with previously. In either case, reviewing the CRF, relevant sections of the protocol that discuss the data being reported, and the specification document (usually a SAP) will give you the foundation you need to review output with an informed eye.

7.3.2 Understanding the Output

In addition to your understanding the data being reported or summarized, it is equally important to have at least a basic understanding of what is being reported. For data listings, this is usually very simple: the data is presented in an easy-to-read, understandable format. However, reviewing this output can require that you check that the correct observations are reported (for example, a data listing title indicating "Safety Evaluable Population" should not include subjects who were not dosed with study medication) or that the columns presented make sense and are presented in a logical order.

When you create summary statistics to report in a table or figure, it is very helpful to have a basic understanding of the statistics being generated. Some of the most common statistics reported are means, medians, and standard deviations. It is critical to understand that the mean and median values should both be between the minimum and maximum values for a given variable; anything else is an obvious error. Similarly, *p*-values are another common statistic that most programmers do not have an intimate understanding of (nor do they need to in order to execute their job effectively). However, it is important to understand that *p*-values should be between 0 and 1. Other summary statistics that are calculated for clinical trials can be unfamiliar to anyone other than a statistician. Although detailed specifications (and even small pieces of code) might be provided, it is important to speak with the originator of these specifications to get an understanding of what a reasonable result for that particular statistic would be. This is the only way to ensure that your review of the output is reasonable, if not correct.

7.3.3 Checking the Result

To ensure that the final data or summary statistics are correct, the techniques described in Chapter 4 should be used throughout the code written to create tables/listings/figures (TLF) output. In cases where you are responsible for independently programming to validate another programmer's output, you should consider using original data rather than analysis data. Particularly when checking data listings, you should refer to the original data wherever possible to ensure that the analysis data being used to generate final output is accurate, as well as the report itself.

After the data and summary statistics are prepared, the final output needs to be reviewed to ensure that the data and summary statistics are accurately represented in the final product. The following are key items to check:

1. No values were truncated.

2. All values are rounded correctly.

3. All numeric data is formatted correctly. Find the minimum and maximum values and check that they are correctly reflected in the output (the log should not indicate that BEST. formats were applied).

7.3.3.1 Checking for Truncation

The easiest way to check for truncation is to find the longest value reported and check that it is reflected in its entirety in the final output. In most cases, it is easy enough to review the final output and recognize truncated values. For example, a value of race that appears as "Black, of African Descen" on a summary table is obviously truncated. However, in data listings where verbatim text fields appear, it is not always obvious when data is truncated. In these cases, it is best to find the record with the longest value in the data and then check the final output. There are a few good options for doing this. For small data sets, it is simple just to open the data set in SAS Viewer and look for the longest value. For larger data sets there are two options: either perform a PROC FREQ on the text field, or build in code to flag the longest record. The PROC FREQ output wraps values and enables you to review the values fairly easily. This technique works well for long text values that are wrapped in the PROC FREQ output (simply find the value that wraps most), but can generate a lot of output. For larger data sets, you might find the technique shown in Example 7.1 more efficient.

Example 7.1

```
data check ;
   set orglib.medhist end=lastrec ;
   length longtxt $200 ;
   retain maxlen 0 longtxt ;
   if maxlen le length(trim(mhcom1)) then
   do ;
      maxlen  = length(trim(mhcom1)) ;
      longtxt = mhcom1 ;
   end ;
   if lastrec then put '>>>> LONGEST TEXT VALUE: >>>> ' inv_no=
patid= longtxt= ;
run ;
```

Output 7.1

```
16          data check ;
17             set orglib.medhist end=lastrec ;
18             length longtxt $200 ;
19             retain maxlen 0 longtxt ;
20             if maxlen le length(trim(mhcom1)) then
21             do ;
22                maxlen  = length(trim(mhcom1)) ;
23                longtxt = mhcom1 ;
24             end ;
25             if lastrec then put '>>>> LONGEST TEXT VALUE: >>>> '
25        ! inv_no= patid= longtxt= ;
26
27          run ;


>>>> LONGEST TEXT VALUE: >>>> INV_NO=4 PATID=228
longtxt=PINCHED NERVE IN (L) FOOT - 1990 - RESOLVED WITH TARSAL TUNN
EL RELEASE SURGERY; MISALIGNED TOES - 1980 - RESOLVED WITH OSTEOTOMY
 (BILATERAL FOOT SURGERY) - 1980; BROKEN (R) WRIST - 1974 - RESOLVED
 WIT
NOTE: There were 2804 observations read from the data set
      ORGLIB.MEDHIST.
NOTE: The data set WORK.CHECK has 2804 observations and 16 variables.

NOTE: DATA statement used (Total process time):
      real time           0.03 seconds
      cpu time            0.03 seconds
```

Although this technique does involve adding a little extra code, it yields the longest value in a given text field without the need to look through over 2800 records or through pages of PROC FREQ output. Once this record is identified, all you need to do is find it in the data listing. If the value is displayed in its entirety, all other shorter values should be completely displayed as well.

It is important to remember that numeric data can be truncated as well. If numbers are calculated and then stored in text fields for reporting purposes, these numbers can be truncated on the final reports. When storing numbers in character fields, make sure that the character fields are long enough to include not only the numbers but all decimal places, negative signs, and any other relevant symbols (dollar signs, percents, greater or less than signs, etc.). As with verbatim text values, before you convert numeric data to character data, a quick PROC MEANS will show the minimum and maximum values and enable you to check those first when validating. If both the minimum and maximum values are displayed correctly, it is fairly safe to assume that all of the numbers in between are displayed correctly as well.

7.3.3.2 Checking for Accurate Rounding

It is important to round data or calculations with the ROUND function rather than through the use of a format. Although the result might look the same at a quick review, formats do not always round correctly. The first place to check for accurate rounding is in cases where the final reported digit is 4, 5, or 6. In these cases, you should review the original data with all of the pre-rounded precision to make sure that the number was actually rounded rather than simply cut off at the last digit. In addition, it is important to check the specification documents for rounding instructions. If the level of precision for reporting data or summary statistics is unclear, be sure to check with the statistician or whoever wrote the specifications.

7.3.3.3 Checking Formats

Formats are routinely applied to data to facilitate reporting. It is critical that the formats applied to data are accurate (1= "male" rather than 1= "female") and long enough (BEST5. rather than BEST3.). Formatted values must be checked against what they represent to ensure that they accurately reflect the data. An entire study could be misinterpreted if the format for drug code were reversed (for example, if 1 were decoded to "active drug" and 2 were decoded to "placebo" when, in fact, the study medication was administered the other way around). User-defined formats are often overlooked in the validation process. It is important to look at the final output with a critical eye to ensure the data makes sense.

To check that formats are long enough to fully report numeric values that include decimal points and negative signs, the first place to look is in the log. If a format that is applied to a variable is not long enough to capture the entire value, SAS usually gives a helpful note stating "NOTE: At least one W.D format was too small for the number to be printed. The decimal may be shifted by the "BEST" format." This note should always be addressed, as it indicates that the format applied to a variable does not allow for the entire value to be presented accurately. Although SAS adjusts to try to get the entire value printed, this adjustment is likely to result in the data being presented oddly. After you look at the log, it is helpful to find the minimum and maximum values for a variable with PROC MEANS or another relevant procedure. If these two values are represented accurately, others should be as well.

7.3.4 Cross-Checking Related Output

When data is reported for clinical trials, there are almost always data listings that are used to support one or more summary tables. It is important to make sure that summary output accurately reflects what is reported in the supportive data listings. If the demographic summary table reports five females in the Placebo dose group, the data listing should reflect the same. Example 7.2 shows a sample demographics table where sex, age, and race are summarized.

Example 7.2

Table 14.1.3 [TDEMO] Summary of Demographics at Baseline - All treated subjects

		Placebo	Pretendopril 10 mg
Subjects Treated		14	15
Sex			
	n	14	15
	Female	5 (35.7%)	61 (75.3%)
	Male	9 (64.3%)	20 (24.7%)
Age (yrs)			
	n	14	15
	Mean	37.8	35.2
	SD	10.7	11.1
	Range	(21,63)	(18,61)
Race			
	n	14	15
	Asian	0	1 (1.2%)
	Black	0	1 (7.4%)
	Caucasian	14 (100.0%)	13 (87.7%)

The listing excerpt (Placebo subjects only) shown in Example 7.3 should reflect the same summary information as the preceding table. In other words, you should be able to identify (and manually count) the five female subjects in the listing that are reported in the table.

Example 7.3

Listing 1 Subject Listing of Demographics All treated subjects				
Treatment Group (mg/kg)	Subject ID	Sex	Race	Age (yrs)
Placebo	001	Female	Caucasian	54
Placebo	004	Female	Caucasian	28
Placebo	007	Male	Caucasian	31
Placebo	009	Male	Caucasian	43
Placebo	014	Male	Caucasian	32
Placebo	016	Female	Caucasian	23
Placebo	021	Male	Caucasian	47
Placebo	022	Female	Caucasian	21
Placebo	025	Male	Caucasian	40
Placebo	027	Female	Caucasian	63
Placebo	034	Male	Caucasian	27
Placebo	036	Male	Caucasian	28
Placebo	038	Male	Caucasian	50
Placebo	042	Male	Caucasian	21

Besides checking summary tables against data listings, checking population counts across different TLFs is also important. Notice in Example 7.2 that the total number of subjects treated is listed in the first row. These same counts should be reflected in all other summary tables with the same population ("all subjects treated"). Although population counts are the most obvious item to cross-check across tables, there are often other counts to check. In some cases, it might be less obvious what numbers need to match. In one table the summary statistics might appear as a column, while in another they might appear across a row. Consider the following series of adverse event tables. The first example is the overall summary of events, and the subsequent tables summarize the data in more detail. The numbers that are followed by callouts indicate which numbers in the first table correspond to the same numbers in subsequent tables.

Example 7.4

Table 14.1
Overview of Adverse Events
Safety Population

	Study Drug, n (%)	
	Drug A **(N=6)**	**Drug B** **(N=4)**
Total Adverse Events	34	43
Subjects with at Least 1 Adverse Event	**5 (83.3)** ❶	**4 (100.0)** ❶
Subjects with at Least 1 Serious Adverse Event	1 (16.7)	0
Highest Severity:		
Mild	**3 (50.0)** ❷	1 (25.0)
Moderate	**1 (16.7)** ❷	1 (25.0)
Severe	**1 (16.7)** ❷	2 (50.0)
Strongest Relationship to Study Medication:		
Not Related	1 (16.7)	0
Unrelated	1 (16.7)	0
Unlikely	0	0
Related ❸	**4 (66.7)** ❸	**4 (100.0)** ❸
Possibly	1 (16.7)	1 (25.0)
Probably	1 (16.7)	0
Definitely	2 (33.3)	3 (75.0)

Example 7.5

Table 14.2

Adverse Events by System Organ Class and Preferred Term

Safety Population

MedDRA SOC Preferred Term	Study Drug, # n (%)a			
	Drug A (N=6)		Drug B (N=4)	
Total Adverse Events	34	**5 (83.3)** **❶**	43	**4 (100.0)** **❶**
GASTROINTESTINAL DISORDERS	14	3 (50.0)	14	4 (100.0)
ABDOMINAL DISCOMFORT	1	1 (16.7)	1	1 (25.0)
ABDOMINAL DISTENSION	0	0	1	1 (25.0)
ABDOMINAL PAIN	2	2 (33.3)	0	0
ABDOMINAL TENDERNESS	0	0	1	1 (25.0)
CONSTIPATION	0	0	2	2 (50.0)
DIARRHOEA	4	3 (50.0)	2	2 (50.0)
DYSPEPSIA	1	1 (16.7)	0	0
FLATULENCE	1	1 (16.7)	0	0

a For each preferred term and System Organ Class: # = number of occurrences; n = number of subjects; % = percentage based on number (N) of safety subjects in each group.

Example 7.6

Table 14.3
Adverse Events by Maximum Severity By Study Group
Safety Population

MedDRA SOC Preferred Term	Study Drug A (N=6), # n (%)a					
	Mild		Moderate		Severe	
Total Adverse Events	24	3 (50.0) ❷	8	1 (16.7) ❷	2	1 (16.7) ❷
GASTROINTESTINAL DISORDERS	11	1 (16.7)	3	2 (33.3)	0	0
ABDOMINAL DISCOMFORT	1	1 (16.7)	0	0	0	0
ABDOMINAL PAIN	1	1 (16.7)	1	1 (16.7)	0	0
DIARRHOEA	3	2 (33.3)	1	1 (16.7)	0	0
DYSPEPSIA	1	1 (16.7)	0	0	0	0
FLATULENCE	1	1 (16.7)	0	0	0	0
GASTROOESOPHAGEAL REFLUX DISEASE	1	1 (16.7)	0	0	0	0
NAUSEA	2	2 (33.3)	0	0	0	0
VOMITING	1	1 (16.7)	1	1 (16.7)	0	0

a For each preferred term and System Organ Class: # = number of occurrences; n = number of subjects; % = percentage based on number (N) of safety subjects in group.

Example 7.7

Table 14.4

Study Medication Related Adverse Events ❸

Safety Population

MedDRA SOC Preferred Term	Study Drug, # n (%)[a]			
	Drug A (N=6)		Drug B (N=4)	
Total Adverse Events	25	**4 (66.7)** ❸	19	**4(100.0)** ❸
GASTROINTESTINAL DISORDERS	14	**3 (50.0)**	10	**4(100.0)**
ABDOMINAL DISCOMFORT	1	1 (16.7)	1	1 (25.0)
ABDOMINAL PAIN	2	2 (33.3)	0	0
ABDOMINAL PAIN UPPER	0	0	1	1 (25.0)
CONSTIPATION	0	0	1	1 (25.0)
DIARRHOEA	4	3 (50.0)	2	2 (50.0)
DYSPEPSIA	1	1 (16.7)	0	0
FLATULENCE	1	1 (16.7)	0	0
GASTROOESOPHAGEAL REFLUX DISEASE	1	1 (16.7)	0	0
NAUSEA	2	2 (33.3)	4	4(100.0)
VOMITING	2	2 (33.3)	1	1 (25.0)

[a] For each preferred term and System Organ Class: # = number of occurrences; n = number of
subjects; % = percentage based on number (N) of safety subjects in each group.

The preceding examples clearly show how the same summary statistics can be reported
across tables in slightly different ways. It is critical to the validation process that programmers understand the output well enough to know what numbers should be the same
across tables, particularly when those similarities are not obvious, as is the case for the
counts in Example 7.7.

7.3.5 Checking the Cosmetics

The review of the cosmetics of the output—reviewing spelling accuracy in row and column headings, reviewing spelling accuracy and correct representation of footnotes, checking that the data layout is neat and consistent, and checking that the overall content matches specifications – is often considered the least important step in the validation process. Before this, all focus has been on the accuracy of the data or statistics being reported in the body of the output, but this step is crucial in making sure that the data is presented clearly. Simple spelling mistakes can undermine the reviewer's confidence in the output as a whole ("If they didn't check spelling, I wonder what else they didn't check?"). Inaccurately represented footnotes can lead to confusion about what the output represents. Poorly presented data can distract the reviewer from the content of the output. Consider the following example, an alternate presentation of Example 7.6.

Example 7.8

Table 14.3

Adverse Events by Maximum Severty By Study Group

Safety Population

MedDRA SOC Preferred Term	Study Drug A (N=6), # n (%)[a]					
	Mild		Moderate		Severe	
Total Adverse Events	24	3 (50.0)	8	1 (16.7)	2	1 (16.7)
GASTROINTESTINAL DISORDERS	11	1 (16.7)	3	2 (33.3)	0	0
ABDOMINAL DISCOMFORT	1	1 (16.7)	0	0	0	0
ABDOMINAL PAIN	1	1 (16.7)	1	1 (16.7)	0	0
DIARRHOEA	3	2 (33.3)	1	1 (16.7)	0	0
DYSPEPSIA	1	1 (16.7)	0	0	0	0
FLATULENCE	1	1 (16.7)	0	0	0	0
GASTROOESOPHAGEAL REFLUX DISEASE	1	1 (16.7)	0	0	0	0
NAUSEA	2	2 (33.3)	0	0	0	0
VOMITING	1	1 (16.7)	1	1 (16.7)	0	0

[a] For each preferred term and System Organ Class: # = number of occurrences; % = percentage based on number (N) of safety subjects in group.

In this example, all of the numbers reported in the table are exactly the same as those reported in the previous table. However, there are several problems with this presentation, starting with the misspelling in the title. In this presentation, the alignment of the columns is inconsistent and the alignment in the first column does not present the data clearly (it is not obvious that the non-bolded terms belong to the bolded category). The alignment of columns also makes it unclear which numbers fall under which column (Mild or Moderate). In addition, a section of the footnote explaining what "n" represents is missing. Although the important part of the output—the data—is correct, the presentation distracts from the actual content, and the omissions can lead to confusion.

The final aspect of reviewing the cosmetics of a table is ensuring that page breaks are consistent and that any data that splits across pages is still represented in its entirety. Consider the following data listing that splits data for a single subject across two pages.

Example 7.9

Page 1 of 2

Listing 4

Adverse Events

Study Drug A

Subject	MeDRA SOC/ MedDRA Preferred Term/ CRF Verbatim Term	Onset Date/ Stop Date/ Duration (days)	Severity
001-002	INVESTIGATIONS	05DEC2007	Mild
	WEIGHT DECREASED	10JAN2007	
	WEIGHT LOSS	37	
	GASTROINTESTINAL DISORDERS	21DEC2006	Mild
	ABDOMINAL DISCOMFORT	24DEC2006	
	ABDOMINAL DISCOMFORT	4	
	GASTROINTESTINAL DISORDERS	25DEC2006	Mild
	DIARRHOEA	30DEC2006	
	LOOSE STOOLS	6	

Listing 4

Adverse Events

Study Drug A

Subject	MedDRA SOC/ MedDRA Preferred Term/ CRF Verbatim Term	Onset Date/ Stop Date/ Duration (days)	Severity
	GASTROINTESTINAL DISORDERS	25DEC2006	Moderate
	NAUSEA	24JAN2007	
	NAUSEA	31	
	GASTROINTESTINAL DISORDERS	01JAN2007	Mild
	DIARRHOEA	04JAN2007	
	DIARRHEA	4	

In the preceding example, there is no indication of which subject these events belong to on the second page. Although it is simple enough in a small example like this to simply turn back to the previous page, in larger examples where a subject's data could span several pages it is time consuming to page back to find the first item for a subject. And if the reviewer is not careful, he or she could miss the subject ID and attribute the events to the wrong subject. One method of resolving this issue is printing the subject ID on every row, but with the duplicate IDs in gray.

Example 7.10

Listing 4
Adverse Events

Study Drug A

Subject	MedDRA SOC/ MedDRA Preferred Term/ CRF Verbatim Term	Onset Date/ Stop Date/ Duration (days)	Severity
001-002	INVESTIGATIONS WEIGHT DECREASED WEIGHT LOSS	05DEC2007 10JAN2007 37	Mild
001-002	GASTROINTESTINAL DISORDERS ABDOMINAL DISCOMFORT ABDOMINAL DISCOMFORT	21DEC2006 24DEC2006 4	Mild
001-002	GASTROINTESTINAL DISORDERS DIARRHOEA LOOSE STOOLS	25DEC2006 30DEC2006 6	Mild

Listing 4
Adverse Events

Study Drug A

Subject	MedDRA SOC/ MedDRA Preferred Term/ CRF Verbatim Term	Onset Date/ Stop Date/ Duration (days)	Severity
001-002	GASTROINTESTINAL DISORDERS NAUSEA NAUSEA	25DEC2006 24JAN2007 31	Moderate
001-002	GASTROINTESTINAL DISORDERS DIARRHOEA DIARRHEA	01JAN2007 04JAN2007 4	Mild

In this example, all of the information needed to correctly interpret the data is present on the second page. It is important to ensure that page breaks do not interfere with the clear presentation of the data.

7.3.6 Updating the Specifications

As programs are being developed, programmers might find data and programming issues that require information additional to that provided in the SAP or other standard specification documents. In most cases, data issues become apparent either when programmers are trying to execute some logic in the code or when they are reviewing the final output. The best source for discovering the source of these data issues is generally someone in the data management department. Such a resource can often shed light on what is happening with the data, such as outstanding queries (requests for clarification or corrections sent to investigational sites for resolution), data problems (missing or erroneous data), or changes in allowed responses (responses that are no longer considered errors). In cases where new responses are now expected to occur in the data, it is important to update the corresponding specifications to include these new values.

In addition to code changes made to handle new data issues, adjustments in how data is presented in the TLFs might also be necessary. Columns or rows might need to be added to tables and listings to accommodate new values occurring in the data. In these cases, the mocks in the SAP should be updated to reflect these changes.

Although programmers should note any data issues that affect how code is written or data is displayed within the program itself, the specification documentation should be updated so that both the original programmer and the validator can work from the same specification. In cases where the code works as it should but the data issue is apparent in the output, it is also helpful to make note of any additional information gathered about the issue in the validation files.

7.3.7 Keeping What Is Important

When validating output, what do you really need to keep? It is recommended that you create a hardcopy validation folder for each type of data collected (one each for subject demographics, medical history, adverse events, etc.). This folder should contain the following:

- A copy of each TLF mock pertaining to that type of data.

- Copies of signed validation checklists and all programs that create output for that type of data. A hard copy of the program as it existed when the validation checklist was signed is recommended in case of any problems with the electronic file, such as the file being lost or modified unintentionally.

- Any correspondence or documentation of decisions made regarding the analysis and reporting of that data type.

When you are deciding what to keep (either as electronic files or on paper), the critical thing to keep in mind is that you need to be able to prove to an independent reviewer that you validated your output per SOP and good practice guidelines.

7.4 Final QC Steps

Most development and validation occurs before receipt of a final database. It is critical that after final data is received, all programs are run and final output is reviewed in its entirety one more time before being delivered to either an internal or external client. Final data updates could result in unforeseen issues in the output that were not present before receipt of final data. All logs must be reviewed for warnings and unanticipated notes, and final output should be reviewed for unexpected data issues. This is also a good chance to make sure output appears consistent across the entire TLF package. Often several programmers are working on a given study, and it is important that the final output looks as though it was produced by one cohesive entity. Although solid specification documentation and SOPs go a long way in ensuring this, there is no substitute for a knowledgeable review of the output.

7.5 Conclusion

The clear and accurate representation of clinical trial data is crucial. Careful and complete validation of summary statistics and other reports generated by programmers is absolutely critical in proving that the results are accurate. This chapter examined the final step of the validation process—validating the final output. Using these methods to validate various types of output will enable you to confidently deliver a validated, high-quality product that accurately represents the study data.

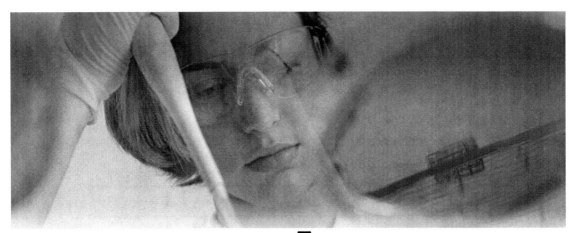

Appendix A

Sample Quality Control Checklists

DERIVED DATA SET PROGRAM VALIDATION QC CHECKLIST

Client: _____   Product: _____

Protocol/Project: _____   Program Name: _____

Program Author: _____

Program Validator: _____   REVIEW / PROGRAM: _____

QUALITY CHECKS	COMPLETED	
Check program log for notes, warning messages, and errors.	A:	Y
	V:	Y
Check program header and comments accurately describe the code.	A:	Y / NA
	V:	Y / NA
Check derived data values against source data for a patient sample to ensure correct derivation.	A:	Y / NA
	V:	Y / NA
Check that all mathematical algorithms specified in the Analysis Plan (AP*) have been implemented correctly.	A:	Y / NA
	V:	Y / NA
Verify that variables needed to support tables/listings/figures are found in the derived data set.	A:	Y / NA
	V:	Y / NA
Check that all formats and subgroups conform to the AP*.	A:	Y / NA
	V:	Y / NA
Check data points for values outside expected ranges, where appropriate.	A:	Y / NA
	V:	Y / NA
Check that data are rounded correctly and in accordance with the AP*.	A:	Y / NA
	V:	Y / NA
Check that data fields are not truncated.	A:	Y / NA
	V:	Y / NA

Program Author Signature: _____   Date: _____

Program Validator Signature: _____   Date: _____

A: Program Author
V: Program Validator
* Or other documents that include relevant project specifications (e.g. protocol, emails, review comments, etc.)

QC CHECKLIST FOR PROGRAMS THAT CONVERT INPUT DATA INTO
FINAL TABLES, LISTINGS, AND FIGURES

Program:_____

QUALITY CHECKS	CHECK COMPLETE	NOT APPLICABLE
• Check program logs for notes, errors, and warning messages		
• Check that the format of the output and all titles and footnotes conform to the mock-ups in the Analysis Plan		
• Check that all abbreviations, range categories, and subgroups conform to the Analysis Plan		
• Check that all data points fully and accurately represent the source data		
• Check that all algorithms specified in the Analysis Plan are implemented correctly		
• Check that all summary statistics are correct; check at least one category in each summary table against the data listings		
• Ensure that data are rounded correctly and in accordance with the Analysis Plan		
• Check all relevant data points for values outside of expected ranges		
• Check that all tables and listings split between pages are done appropriately and consistently		
• Check that there are no columns completely blank unless appropriate and that there are no duplicate rows		
• Check that data fields are not truncated or run together		
• Ensure the consistency of population counts across relevant tables, listings, and figures		

Signature:_____   Date:_____

Project ID: _____

Programmer Name: _____

QC Programmer: _____

Program Name / Output Generated	Comments	Comments	Comments	Comments	Comments
Date Reviewed, Initials					
Standard program/file/directory naming conventions used					
If the program produces output					
Output format consistent with client request *					
No typo's, misspellings or nonsensical values in output					
Cross-checked similar data types across tables, figures and listings					
Number of observations correct for patient population					
All programs					
Standard variable / dataset naming conventions used					
Standard header used, includes documentation of program modifications					
Programming style guidelines have been followed **					
Verification code supplied before and after selected data processing steps					
Data manipulation/calculation fields checked					
Data handling specifications applied correctly					
Date and time of program execution present on all log and output files					
Log is free of errors, warnings and other messages that may suggest syntactic or logic problems ***					
Log has accurate and consistent variable counts					

* As documented in analysis plan and comments on previous outputs

** Programming style guidelines may be modified per client needs/specifications

*** Log is attached. Any questionable messages remaining in the log must be explained/justified in comments area.

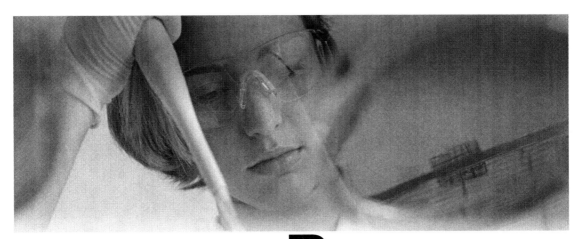

Appendix B

Sample Statistical Analysis Plan

STATISTICAL ANALYSIS PLAN

Title: A 6-Week, Double-Blind, Placebo-Controlled, Randomized, Multicenter Study of the Safety and Efficacy of 6 and 12 mg/day Pretendopril Doses for the Treatment of Headaches

Protocol: ABC-123

Study Drug: PRETENDOPRIL

Sponsor: Example Pharmaceutical, Inc.

Author: Joe Statistician

Date: January 10, 2006

Status: FINAL

Approved by:

Example Pharmaceutical Inc.:   _____   **Date:** _____

TABLE OF CONTENTS OF THE SAP

A 6-Week, Double-Blind, Placebo-Controlled, Randomized, Multicenter Study of the Safety and Efficacy of 6 and 12 mg/day Pretendopril Doses for the Treatment of Headaches

1. STUDY OBJECTIVES

- To evaluate the safety and efficacy compared to placebo of 6 weeks treatment with 6 or 12 mg/day Pretendopril in patients diagnosed with headaches

2. STUDY DESIGN

This was a 6-week, double-blind, placebo-controlled, randomized, multicenter study to evaluate the safety and efficacy of two doses of Pretendopril compared to placebo in the treatment of outpatients with headaches. The two fixed doses of Pretendopril tested were 6 and 12 mg/day. The study was conducted at 4 investigative sites in the United States.

This study was conducted in patients between 18 and 70 years of age with a current episode of headaches of >4 weeks and ≤ 6 months in duration. All patients received single-blind placebo for 1 week (± 3days) during the Screening and Baseline Periods. During this period eligibility criteria were confirmed. Patients meeting these key eligibility criteria along with the other inclusion/exclusion criteria were eligible for randomization once all other baseline tests had been completed.

In the Treatment Period, patients were randomized to receive either 6 or 12 mg/day of Pretendopril or to placebo in a 1:1:1 ratio. Dosing commenced the morning after the day randomized. Randomized study medication was to be taken once daily for 6 weeks.

3. STUDY EVALUATIONS

The study evaluation schedule is summarized in Table A.

Example Pharmaceuticals, Inc. FINAL SAP
ABC-123 10JAN2006

Table A
Study Evaluation Schedule

Assessment	Screening Initial+ Visit	Day -8	Day -1*	End of Week: (+/- 3 days)* Double Blind Treatment 1	2	3	4	5	6^
Written informed consent	X	X							
Inclusion and exclusion criteria		X							
Medical and headache history		X							
Physical Exam		X							X
Vital signs		X	X	X	X	X	X	X	X
Clinical labs (CBC, chem., U/A)		X		X		X			X
Serum Pregnancy Test%		X							X
ECG		X		X					X
Efficacy Test 1		X	X	X	X	X	X	X	X
Efficacy Test 2				X	X	X	X	X	X
Adverse Events			X	X	X	X	X	X	X
Concomitant Medication		X	X	X	X	X	X	X	X
Final eligibility assessment and randomization			X						
Dispense Drug		X	X	X	X	X	X	X	

+ All patients will be seen at an Initial Visit, when written informed consent is obtained. Patients on prohibited headache medication who need to be discontinued will be given explicit instructions for this procedure and will return at Day –8. Patients who do not require discontinuation from prohibited headache medications can be seen for the first time at Day –8. For these patients, the Initial Visit and the Day –8 visit occur simultaneously.

* It is important to maintain the visit structure as accurately as possible. In the rare case in which an adjustment to this structure is necessary, the visit should occur within 3 days of the planned schedule. The timing of subsequent visits should be planned to maintain the visit structure relative to the first day double-blind medication was taken.

^ The Week 6 visit will serve as the End-of-Treatment visit for all patients randomized to treatment in the study. This visit will occur when patients complete the 6-week treatment period or when they terminate treatment prematurely.

% Women of childbearing potential

Example Pharmaceuticals, Inc.   FINAL SAP
ABC-123   10JAN2006

3.1 Demographic and Baseline Characteristics

The following events and clinical observations were obtained during the Screening and Baseline Periods between Day –8 and Day –1.

- Demographic characteristics (Day –8)
- Medical history (Day –8)
- Headache History (Day –8)
- Sitting Vital Signs (Day –8 and Day –1)
- Body Weight and Height (Day –8)
- Physical exam (Day –8)
- Concomitant medications (Day –8 and Day –1)
- 12-Lead Electrocardiogram (Day –8)
- Clinical laboratory tests (Day –8)
- Efficacy Test 1 (Day –8 and Day –1)
- Efficacy Test 2 (Day –8 and Day –1)
- Adverse Events (from Day –8 to Day –1)
- Pregnancy test (Day –8)

3.2 Efficacy Evaluations

Efficacy data consisted of the Efficacy Test 1 and Efficacy Test 2 scores.

Efficacy Test 1

The Efficacy Test 1 questionnaire consisted of 14 separate items each scored between 0–4 with higher scores representative of a more serious state. The questionnaire was completed by the investigator at Day –8, Day –1, Week 1, Week 2, Week 3, Week 4, Week 5 and Week 6. Change in the total score of the 14 items from Day –1 was of interest.

Efficacy Test 2

The Efficacy Test 2 – Overall Improvement Score was recorded at Week 1, Week 2, Week 3, Week 4, Week 5 and Week 6. It was scored on the following seven point scale:

1=Very much improved
2=Much improved
3=Minimally improved
4=No Change
5=Minimally worse
6=Much worse
7=Very much worse

Scores recorded at each visit represented the status of the patient's headache symptoms compared to the Day −1 visit.

3.3 Safety Evaluations

Assessment of safety included:

- Physical examinations

- Vital signs and Body Weight

- 12-Lead Electrocardiogram

- Clinical laboratory tests

- Adverse events

4. STATISTICAL METHODS AND DETERMINATION OF SAMPLE SIZE

All patients randomized and receiving at least one dose of active study drug or placebo control were included in the safety analyses. Two populations were defined for the efficacy analyses. For the primary assessment of efficacy, an "Efficacy Evaluable" population was defined which consisted of patients who met predefined "Key Criteria". An "Intent-to-Treat" population was also defined and included patients who received at least one dose of double-blind medication and had at least one post-baseline value for either Efficacy Test for which a baseline also existed.

All statistical hypothesis tests comparing each dose of Pretendopril vs Placebo were conducted at alpha=0.10 (two-sided). No adjustments for multiple comparisons were employed.

4.1 Data Handling

For the purposes of data listings and summaries which used actual "relative time", time was calculated relative to the first dose of double-blind medication which was considered to be the day immediately following the "Day –1 Visit". The relative day of study medication on the day of dosing was considered as "Day 1". The day prior to the first dose of double-blind study medication was considered as "Day –1". There was no "Day 0".

Efficacy

For the Efficacy Test 1 Score and Efficacy Test 2 score, baseline was defined as the value recorded on Day –1 visit.

Data were summarized using scheduled visits. In addition to the scheduled visits, an endpoint visit was defined by carrying forward the last measurement (Last Visit) recorded after the baseline.

Safety

In general, safety data were summarized according to scheduled visit. Adverse event summaries included all patients receiving at least one dose of double-blind medication. Data other than adverse events were summarized for all patients receiving at least one dose of double-blind medication according to scheduled visit.

Baseline values were selected as the last measurement recorded prior to double-blind dosing. Data collected after the last dose of double-blind medication + 1 day were not included in the summary tables but were included in the data listings. In addition to the scheduled visits, a Last Visit was defined by carrying forward the last measurement (Last Visit) recorded after the baseline and on or before the last dose of double-blind medication + 1 day. If applicable, repeat or unscheduled laboratory values were not included in the summary tables nor were they eligible for last visit carried forward.

To allow differentiation as to which study period an Adverse Event occurred, three categories were defined based upon onset date. Adverse Events which had onset dates prior to the day of first dose of double-blind medication were considered "prior". Adverse events starting on the day of or after the first dose of double-blind medication and before the last dose of double-blind medication + 1 day for non-serious or before the last dose of double-blind medication + 30 days for serious events were considered "on-therapy". Events occurring after this time were considered as "post-therapy" and were listed but not included in the summary tables. If applicable, adverse events with missing onset dates were counted as having occurred "on-therapy". Events that were indicated as "Probably

Study Drug Related", "Possibly Study Drug Related" or had a missing relationship were considered as "Related".

Medications taken any time prior to the first dose of double-blind medication were counted as prior medications. Those taken after the first dose of double-blind medication and before the last dose of double-blind medication + 1 day were counted as concomitant medications. Medications received after the last dose of double-blind medication + 1 day were counted as post-therapy and were not included in summary tables. Medications could be counted in more than one category.

4.2 Efficacy Analysis

The efficacy analyses were conducted on both Intent-to-Treat and Evaluable Patients. Prior to breaking the study blind, patients with violations of selected criteria were identified. Patients with the following protocol violations were identified; however, such violations were not used as a basis to exclude patients from the Evaluable population.

- Efficacy Test 1 total score <20 or >30 at either Day –8 visit or Day –1 visit

- Efficacy Test 2 Score < 4 at either Day –8 visit or Day –1 visit

4.3 Safety Analysis

Analysis of Safety data was performed using the data from all patients who had received at least one dose of the study agent; this was referred to as the safety population.

Adverse Events

Adverse events were coded using the MedDRA dictionary and were categorized by organ class. Unique CRF verbatim terms and the MedDRA preferred terms and organ classes assigned were listed in a matching chart.

On-therapy treatment emergent adverse events were summarized by MedDRA organ class and preferred term as well as by severity (mild, moderate, severe) and by relationship to study medication (related, not related). Summaries counted multiple occurrences of events within a patient as well as patients with at least one occurrence.

Vital Signs

The number of patients who developed changes from baseline of potential clinical significance at any timepoint subsequent to baseline were tabulated and flagged in the patient data listings. Criteria used were as follows:

- Systolic BP: >180 mmHg and an increase of ≥20 mmHg
  < 90 mmHg and a decrease of ≥20 mmHg

- Diastolic BP: >105 mmHg and an increase of ≥15 mmHg
  <50 mmHg and a decrease of ≥15 mmHg

- Pulse Rate: >120 bpm and an increase of ≥15 bpm
  <50 bpm and a decrease of ≥15 bpm

- Body Weight: Decrease of ≥5%

12-Lead Electrocardiogram

The number of patients with values of potential clinical significance at any on-therapy timepoint subsequent to baseline were tabulated and flagged in the patient data listings. Criteria used were as follows:

- PR interval: ≥ 250 msec
- QRS interval: ≥ 150 msec
- QTc interval: ≥ 500 msec

Laboratory Evaluations

Hematology, blood chemistry and continuous urinalysis parameters were summarized using descriptive statistics at each scheduled timepoint and Last Visit according to treatment group. Categorical urinalysis data were tabulated using the number of patients with at least one abnormal value recorded post-baseline according to treatment group and baseline category.

Laboratory data were also evaluated using standard reference ranges from the local and central clinical laboratories to tabulate the occurrence of values above and below the normal reference range as well as using sponsor-defined criteria for changes of potential clinical significance. Patients were tabulated according to their "worst" (i.e. Below or

Above the reference range) on-therapy value. Should a patient have had both a below normal and an above normal value that patient was counted twice in the analysis (one "Low" and one "High") and a footnote documenting the occurrence was provided. All values outside the normal range and changes of potential clinical significance were flagged in the patient data listings.

5. STATISTICAL SOFTWARE

All data summaries and listings were performed using The SAS System®, Version 9.1, or later under Windows operating system.

PROGRAMMING SPECIFICATIONS

1. Required margins: at least 1.5 inches on the binding margin and at least 1 inch on all other sides and minimum 9 pt font. All output should have the following header at the upper left margin:

    Example Pharmaceutical, Inc.
    ABC-123

    And the following header at the upper right margin:

    Page Number (Page n of N)
    Date (ddmmmyyyy)

    All output should have the date (date output was generated) and internal page number at the top right corner. Tables/appendices/listings should be internally paginated (i.e., page numbers should appear sequentially within each table). The name of the SAS program used to generate the output shall be displayed in the lower left corner.

2. Data will be centered within columns when the maximum length of the data being displayed is less than or equal to the maximum width of the column heading. When the maximum length of the data being displayed exceeds the maximum width of the column heading, the data will be left justified. Column headings should be in initial capital characters. Each page of the tables and listings will have an overline at the top to represent the start of data for the page and an underline at the bottom to represent the end of data for that particular page. For numeric variables, include "unit" in the column heading when appropriate.

3. Unless otherwise specified, footnotes should appear on all pages within the table.

PROGRAMMING SPECIFICATIONS (cont'd)

4. Unless otherwise noted, the mean and standard deviation of a set of values should be printed out to one more decimal than the original value.

> e.g., original: xx
> mean and standard deviation: xx.x and xx.x
> range (minimum and maximum): xx, xx

5. All table percentages should be reported with one decimal point unless otherwise noted.

6. Missing data should be represented on patient listings as 1) dashes "-", and properly footnoted: " - = data not available" or 2) "N/A", with footnote "N/A" = not applicable", whichever is appropriate.

7. The following specifications apply to tables that summarize categorical data:

    □ Percent of events should be left blank (including the parentheses) if the number of events is zero.

    □ If the categories of a parameter are ordered, then all categories between the maximum possible category and the minimum category should be included, even if n=0 for a given category between the minimum and maximum level for that parameter.

    □ If the categories are not ordered, then only those categories for which there is at least one Patient represented should be included.

    □ A Missing category should be added to any parameter for which information is not available for any Patients.

8. Relative Study Day

    The day of the study agent administration is Day 1. A (–) sign indicates days prior to the start of study agent (e.g. Day –5 means 5 days prior to administration of study agent; there will be no Day '0').

9. The following algorithm should be used to estimate the start and stop dates of concomitant medications for which only partial information is known:

If only the day is missing, use the first day of the month. If the month and day are missing and the start year is the same as the study year, use <-01:000 (year: day). If the month and day are missing and the start year is prior to the study year, present the number of years only (e.g., –04:000).

If a date is estimated on the patient data listing, it should be flagged and footnoted dynamically as follows:

Estimated date: first day of the month was used if only the day was missing; <-01:000 is indicated if month and day were missing and start year was the study year; number of years only is indicated if month and day were missing and start year was prior to the study year.

10. In general, patient data listings should include all patients with data. However, if a patient data listing includes only patients who met a certain condition, i.e., patients with serious adverse events, and there are no patients who met that condition, then a page marker will appear indicating that no patients met the condition for inclusion.

LIST OF TABLES

Example Pharmaceuticals, Inc.   FINAL SAP
ABC-123   10JAN2006

Efficacy

Table 15.1	Descriptive Statistics for Efficacy Test 1 Total Score
Table 15.2	Analysis of Change in Efficacy Test 1 Total Score at Each Visit
Table 15.3	Descriptive Statistics for Efficacy Test 1—Overall Improvement Score
Table 15.4	Analysis of Efficacy Test 1—Overall Improvement Score

Safety

Table 16.1	Summary of Treatment Emergent Adverse Events
Preface A	MedDRA System Organ Class/Preferred Term and CRF Verbatim Terms
Table 16.2.1	Treatment Emergent Adverse Events by System Organ Class
Table 16.2.2	Treatment Emergent Adverse Events by System Organ Class and Preferred Term
Table 16.3	Treatment Emergent Adverse Events by System Organ Class, Preferred Term and Severity
Table 16.4	Treatment Emergent Adverse Events by System Organ Class, Preferred Term and Relationship to Study Medication
Table 16.5	List of Serious Adverse Events
Table 16.6	List of Adverse Events Leading to Discontinuation
Table 16.7	List of Deaths
Table 17.1	Descriptive Statistics for Vital Signs; Sitting Systolic Blood Pressure (mm Hg)
Table 17.2	Descriptive Statistics for Vital Signs; Sitting Diastolic Blood Pressure (mm Hg)
Table 17.3	Descriptive Statistics for Vital Signs; Sitting Pulse (bpm)
Table 17.4	Descriptive Statistics for Vital Signs; Body Weight (kg)
Table 17.5	Descriptive Statistics for Vital Signs; Temperature (Degree C)
Table 17.6	Descriptive Statistics for Vital Signs; Respiration Rate (per minute)
Table 17.7	Vital Sign Changes of Potential Clinical Significance
Table 17.8	List of Patients with Vital Signs Changes of Potential Clinical Significance
Table 18.1	ECG Values of Potential Clinical Significance
Table 18.2	List of Patients with ECG Values of Potential Clinical Significance

LABORATORY DATA
Summary Statistics for Hematology Laboratory Parameters

Summary Statistics for Blood Chemistry Laboratory Parameters

Urinalysis

Example Pharmaceuticals, Inc.   FINAL SAP
ABC-123   10JAN2006

PATIENT DATA LISTINGS

Clinical Laboratory Values by Parameter

Note: Only two mocks are provided in this appendix—an actual SAP would contain
mocks for each unique table or listing format noted in the table of contents.

Example Pharmaceutical, Inc.
ABC-123

Table 14.1

Demographic and Baseline Characteristics

Study Population: Safety

Characteristic	Placebo (N=xx)	6 mg (N=xx)	12 mg (N=xx)	Total (N=xx)
Gender n(%)				
Male	xx (x.x)	xx (x.x)	xx (x.x)	xx (x.x)
Female	xx (x.x)	xx (x.x)	xx (x.x)	xx (x.x)
Age (yrs)				
[N] mean (SD)	[xx] xx.x (xx.x)	[xx] xx.x (xx.x)	[xx] xx.x (xx.x)	[xx] xx.x (xx.x)
n (%)				
18-39	xx (x.x)	xx (x.x)	xx (x.x)	xx (x.x)
40-64	xx (x.x)	xx (x.x)	xx (x.x)	xx (x.x)
>=65	xx (x.x)	xx (x.x)	xx (x.x)	xx (x.x)
Race n(%)				
White	xx (x.x)	xx (x.x)	xx (x.x)	xx (x.x)
Black	xx (x.x)	xx (x.x)	xx (x.x)	xx (x.x)
Asian	xx (x.x)	xx (x.x)	xx (x.x)	xx (x.x)
Other	xx (x.x)	xx (x.x)	xx (x.x)	xx (x.x)
Weight* (kg)				
[N] mean (SD)	[xx] xx.x (xx.x)	[xx] xx.x (xx.x)	[xx] xx.x (xx.x)	[xx] xx.x (xx.x)
Height (cm)				
[N] mean (SD)	[xx] xx.x (xx.x)	[xx] xx.x (xx.x)	[xx] xx.x (xx.x)	[xx] xx.x (xx.x)

* Last measurement prior to dosing with double-blind medication.

Example Pharmaceutical, Inc.
ABC-123

Listing 1.1

Demographic and Baseline Characteristics

Center/ Patient	Age (yrs)	Gender	Race	Weight* (kg)	Height (cm)
Treatment = Placebo					
		Male Female	Caucasian Black Asian Hispanic American Indian or Specify Other		

---

* Last measurement recorded prior to dosing with double-blind medication.

Footnote "- = data not available" whenever appropriate.

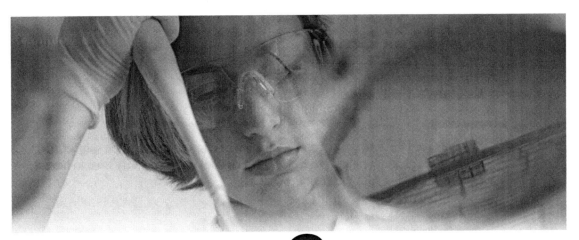

Appendix C

Glossary

aCRF

See annotated case report form.

ADaM

See analysis dataset model.

adverse event

Any untoward medical occurrence in a patient or clinical investigation subject administered a pharmaceutical product and which does not necessarily have to have a causal relationship with this treatment. (ICH)

AE

See adverse event.

analysis dataset model

An organized collection of data or information with a common theme arranged in rows and columns and represented as a single file; comparable to a database table. Note: Standardizing analysis datasets is intended to make review and assessment of analysis more consistent.

analysis data, analysis data set

Data sets created to support specific analyses. (www.fda.gov/cder/regulatory/ersr/ Studydata.pdf)

annotated case report form

A printed or electronic case report form with the data set and variable names that correspond to every unique item on each page written or recorded on the page.

archive area

An area where older versions of data and/or programs are stored.

audit

A systematic and independent examination of trial related activities and documents to determine whether the evaluated trial related activities were conducted, and the data were recorded, analyzed and accurately reported according to the protocol, sponsor's standard operating procedures (SOPs), Good Clinical Practice (GCP), and the applicable regulatory requirement(s). (ICH)

audit trail

Documentation that allows reconstruction of the course of events. (ICH)

blind, blinding

1) Data or reports where the treatment assignment for each subject is not known or revealed; 2) a procedure in which one or more parties to the trial are kept unaware of the treatment assignment(s). (ICH)

case report form

A printed, optical, or electronic document designed to record all of the protocol required information to be reported to the sponsor on each trial subject. (ICH)

CDISC

See Clinical Data Interchange Standards Consortium.

cell index

Output generated by PROC PRINT using both the BY and ID statements to create a grouped listing with all of the individual records contributing to any specific statistic (cell) on a summary table.

centralized laboratory

A single laboratory facility to which all blood, urine, or other biological samples from subjects in a clinical trial are sent for analysis. Can also refer to facilities that analyze specific types of data collected for all subjects in a clinical trial (for example, ECG data or x-ray images).

CFR

See Code of Federal Regulations.

change control

The method and documentation by which changes to an original document, program, or data are tracked from a given point to final archival.

Clinical Data Interchange Standards Consortium

A team of industry professionals, including members from the FDA, whose mission is "to develop and support global, platform-independent data standards that enable information system interoperability to improve medical research and related areas of healthcare." (www.cdisc.org)

clinical trial report / clinical study report

A written description of a trial/study of any therapeutic, prophylactic, or diagnostic agent conducted in human subjects, in which the clinical and statistical description, presentations, and analyses are fully integrated into a single report. (ICH)

COBRA

See Consolidated Omnibus Budget Reconciliation Act.

Code of Federal Regulations

The codification of the general and permanent rules published by the Federal Register by the executive departments and agencies of the Federal Government. (www.gpoaccess.gov/cfr/index.html)

common toxicity criteria

A grading system used to determine the severity of an adverse event or laboratory test result.

compliance

Adherence to all the trial-related requirements, Good Clinical Practice requirements, and applicable regulatory requirements. (ICH)

Consolidated Omnibus Budget Reconciliation Act

An act that gives workers and their families who lose their health benefits the right to choose to continue group health benefits provided by their group health plan for limited periods of time under certain circumstances. (www.dol.gov/dol/topic/health-plans/cobra.htm)

contract research organization

A person or an organization (commercial, academic, or other) contracted by the sponsor to perform one or more of a sponsor's trial-related duties and functions. (ICH)

CRF

See case report form.

CRO

See contract research organization.

CTC

See common toxicity criteria.

CTR / CSR

See clinical trial report / clinical study report.

data definition table

A document that describes the format and content of data sets submitted to regulatory authorities. Specifications for exactly what these files should contain are detailed in various FDA and CDISC guidelines.

data management

The department of individuals responsible for collecting clinical trial data and reviewing that data to ensure it follows protocol and CRF completion guidelines, as well as making basic clinical sense.

data tabulations

Data sets in which each record is a single observation for a subject. (www.fda.gov/cder/regulatory/ersr/Studydata.pdf)

DDT

See data definition table.

demographics/demography

General subject information including (but not limited to) sex, race, and date of birth.

Department of Health and Human Services

A cabinet department of the United States government with the goal of protecting the health of all Americans and providing essential human services. (www.hhs.gov/about/whatwedo.html)

derived data, derived variable

Data sets/variables that are manipulated or derived from original data sources for reporting or summary purposes.

DHHS

See Department of Health and Human Services.

dirty data

Data with issues such as inconsistent data (height is reported as 200 inches while weight is reported as 65 pounds), unexpected values, and/or missing data.

disposition

Information regarding how a subject completed a clinical trial or stage of a clinical trial, and if they did not complete, the reason(s) why.

documentation

Information and documents that programmers work with as well as what programmers provide.

domain (data)

A collection of logically related observations with a topic-specific commonality about the subjects in the trial. (CDISC--Study Data Tabulation Model Implementation Guide: Human Clinical Trials version 3.1.1)

ECG

Electrocardiogram.

eCTD

See electronic Common Technical Document.

efficacy

Evidence that the study treatment has an effect on subjects.

electronic Common Technical Document

The format in which all data and documents collected during the development process (including clinical trials) is submitted to the FDA; ICH defines this as "an interface for industry to agency transfer of regulatory information." (http://estri.ich.org/eCTD/eCTD_Specification_v3_2.pdf)

FDA

See Food and Drug Administration.

first-level validation, first-round validation

Performed by a programmer during development of the production programming suite.

follow-up period

The time after study treatment has been completed when subjects are followed to collect additional safety, efficacy, and/or survival information.

Food and Drug Administration

An agency of the United States Department of Health and Human Services and is responsible for the safety regulation of most types of foods, dietary supplements, drugs, vaccines, biological medical products, blood products, medical devices, radiation-emitting devices, veterinary products, and cosmetics. (www.fda.gov/opacom/morechoices/mission.html)

GCP

See good clinical practice.

good clinical practice

A standard for the design, conduct, performance, monitoring, auditing, recording, analyses, and reporting of clinical trials that provides assurance that the data and reported results are credible and accurate, and that the rights, integrity, and confidentiality of trial subjects are protected. (ICH)

hard-code

A method of changing the value and meaning of a data point through the use of a program outside of a CFR Part 11-compliant data management system (changing the data without the use of an approved audit trail).

Health Insurance Portability and Accountability Act of 1996

Title I of HIPAA protects health insurance coverage for workers and their families when they change or lose their jobs. Title II of HIPAA, the Administrative Simplification (AS) provisions, requires the establishment of national standards for electronic health care transactions and national identifiers for providers, health insurance plans, and employers. (www.hhs.gov/ocr/hipaa)

HIPAA

See Health Insurance Portability and Accountability Act of 1996.

ICH

See International Conference on Harmonisation of Technical Requirements for Registration of Pharmaceuticals for Human Use.

impute (data)

A method of assigning a value for a missing data point that is usually based on another related data point.

independent programming

The process where two different programmers create output and then compare the finished results.

informed consent

A process by which a subject voluntarily confirms his or her willingness to participate in a particular trial, after having been informed of all aspects of the trial that are relevant to the subject's decision to participate. Informed consent is documented by means of a written, signed, and dated informed consent form. (ICH)

intent-to-treat population

Usually includes any subject who agreed to participate in the trial (by signing an informed consent form) and who was officially included in the trial (usually by being assigned a study ID and treatment).

International Conference on Harmonisation of Technical Requirements for Registration of Pharmaceuticals for Human Use

A unique project that brings together the regulatory authorities of Europe, Japan and the United States and experts from the pharmaceutical industry in the three regions to discuss scientific and technical aspects of product registration. The purpose is to make recommendations on ways to achieve greater harmonisation in the interpretation and application of technical guidelines and requirements for product registration. (www.ich.org)

key identifiers

The minimum variables needed to identify a single, unique record in a data set.

laboratory tests

Any of a variety of tests run on blood and/or urine samples (such as glucose and cholesterol tests).

local laboratory

A laboratory facility that is local to each investigative site or subject in a clinical trial to which blood, urine, or other biological samples are sent for analysis.

Medical Dictionary for Regulated Activities

An electronic dictionary that is used to categorize adverse events. (www.meddramsso.com/MSSOWeb/index.htm)

MedDRA

See Medical Dictionary for Regulated Activities.

mock-up, mock, shell

A representation of what each unique table, listing or figure should look like in the final reports but without any values present (essentially, report titles, column and row headings, and footnotes laid out on a page as the author would like them to appear).

National Cancer Institute

Part of the United States Federal Government's National Institutes of Health. The NCI is a federally funded research and development center, one of eight agencies that compose the Public Health Service in the United States Department of Health and Human Services and is the Federal Government's principal agency for cancer research and training. (www.cancer.gov/aboutnci/overview/mission)

NCI

See National Cancer Institute.

NDA

See New Drug Application.

New Drug Application

A vehicle through which drug sponsors formally propose that the FDA approve a new pharmaceutical for sale and marketing in the United States. (www.fda.gov/cder/regulatory/applications/NDA.htm)

normalized data

Data wherein duplication of information is minimized.

one-off program

A unique program that is written to perform one specific function.

original data / raw data

Data as it is first received from the data collection database (or other source) for analysis and reporting purposes.

peer review

A process wherein one programmer programs output, then another programmer reviews the code to ensure that the code and output are correct.

predicate rules

Any requirements listed under CFR Title 21.

production code, production program

A program that creates the final output that is delivered by programming.

programming guidelines

One or more documents that contain a detailed set of instructions for programmers to follow to maintain a consistent program structure and methodology for performing common tasks.

protocol

A document that describes the objective(s), design, methodology, statistical consider-ations, and organization of a trial. (ICH)

QA

See quality assurance.

QC

See quality control.

quality assurance

All those planned and systematic actions that are established to ensure that the trial is performed and the data are generated, documented (recorded), and reported in compliance with Good Clinical Practice (GCP) and the applicable regulatory requirement(s). (ICH)

quality control

The operational techniques and activities undertaken within the quality assurance system to verify that the requirements for quality of the trial-related activities have been fulfilled. (ICH)

randomization

The process of assigning trial subjects to treatment or control groups using an ele-ment of chance to determine the assignments in order to reduce bias. (ICH)

randomization data set

The data set that contains subjects treatment group assignments.

RBC

Red blood cells.

reconcile (variables)

A process that compares the values of similar variables from two different sources to make sure that they are the same.

safety data

Any data collected on the CRF that demonstrates whether the study treatment is safe or not. Generally this data includes adverse events, vital signs, laboratory test, and physical exam results.

safety population

A group that generally includes any subject who received at least one study treatment (drug or procedure) during a clinical trial.

SAP

See statistical analysis plan.

SDLC

See software development life cycle.

SDTM

See Study Data Tabulation Model.

second-level validation, second round validation

A process wherein a programmer who did not write the original programming code to create the output, writes code independently, then the results of the two sets of code are compared and reconciled.

software

Programs, procedures, rules, and any associated documentation pertaining to the operation of a system. (http://www.fda.gov/ora/inspect_ref/igs/gloss.html)

software development life cycle

The process that is followed and documented from the start of the programming process through to final code development and maintenance.

SOP

See standard operating procedures.

sponsor

An individual, company, institution, or organization that takes responsibility for the initiation, management, and/or financing of a clinical trial. (ICH)

Standard International units (SI units)

A global standard for reporting laboratory results, which are usually metric.

standard operating procedures

Detailed, written instructions to achieve uniformity of the performance of a specific function. (ICH)

statistical analysis plan

A document that defines the statistical analyses that will be performed for the clinical trial and details all of the summary tables, data listings, and figures that will need to be generated to report those analyses.

Study Data Tabulation Model

A set of CDISC standards for submitting data tabulations.

study/subject ID

A unique identifier assigned by the investigator to each trial subject to protect the subject's identity and used in lieu of the subject's name when the investigator reports adverse events and/or other trial related data. (ICH)

subject/trial subject

An individual who participates in a clinical trial, either as a recipient of the investigational product(s) or as a control. (ICH)

tables, listings, and figures

Typical output for analysis of clinical trial data and for submission to regulatory agencies. Tables are typically summaries of the data; listings are lists of data that are included in the summaries. Figures are graphical representations of the data being analyzed.

TLFs

See tables, listings, and figures.

traceability

The ability to chronologically follow changes in data or programs from a starting to finishing point.

unblind, unblinding

A process by which the treatment assignment (study drug/procedure) that each study subject received is revealed or reported.

validation

A justification of the means used to accomplish the outcome of a program and its accurate representation of the original data.

validation checklists

Checklists that list the items that must be reviewed and approved during the validation process. These checklists usually require the person performing the checks to initial or sign and date the checklist when it is completed for each item (data set, table, etc.) being validated.

validation output

Output that is created solely for validation purposes (will not be presented formally).

validation programmer

The programmer who is responsible for second-level validation.

validation programs

Programs that are created during second-level validation to validate production programming.

verification

Confirmation of the system and the data accuracy.

WBC

White blood cells.

WHODRL

See World Health Organization Drug Reference List.

World Health Organization Drug Reference List

An electronic dictionary that is used to categorize medications.

Note: Definitions provided by the International Conference on Harmonisation Guidelines for Good Clinical Practice (http://www.ich.org/LOB/media/MEDIA482.pdf) are designated by (ICH).

References

American Psychological Association (APA): software. Dictionary.com Unabridged (v 1.1). Random House, Inc. http://dictionary.reference.com/browse/software

Chicago Manual Style (CMS): software. Dictionary.com Unabridged (v 1.1). Random House, Inc. http://dictionary.reference.com/browse/software

Code of Federal Regulations, Title 21, Volume 8; cite 21CFR820.70

Federal Register, 21 CFR Part 11 – Subpart B §11.10 (e)

http://estri.ich.org/eCTD/eCTD_Specification_v3_2.pdf

International Conference on Harmonisation of Technical Requirements for Registration of Pharmaceuticals for Human Use, "ICH Harmonised Tripartite Guideline, Guide line for Good Clinical Practice, E6(R1), Current Step 4 version." Dated 10 June 1996. (www.ich.org/LOB/media/MEDIA482.pdf)

Modern Language Association (MLA): software. Dictionary.com Unabridged (v 1.1). Random House, Inc. http://dictionary.reference.com/browse/software

"Study Data Tabulation Model Implementation Guide: Human Clinical Trials." Prepared by the CDISC Submission Data Standards Team. CDISC: Copyright © 2005. Dated August 26, 2005.

www.cancer.gov/aboutnci/overview/mission

www.cdisc.org

www.cdisc.org/glossary/V6_Glossary2007.pdf

www.dol.gov/dol/topic/health-plans/cobra.htm

www.fda.gov/cber/gdlns/elecgen.htm

www.fda.gov/cder/guidance/7087rev.htm

www.fda.gov/cder/guidance/959fnl.pdf

www.fda.gov/cder/guidance/ICH_E9-fnl.pdf

www.fda.gov/cder/regulatory/applications/NDA.htm

www.fda.gov/cder/regulatory/ersr/Studydata.pdf

www.fda.gov/opacom/morechoices/mission.html

www.fda.gov/ora/inspect_ref/igs/gloss.html

www.gpoaccess.gov/cfr/index.html

www.hhs.gov/about/whatwedo.html

www.hhs.gov/ocr/hipaa

www.ich.org

www.labcompliance.com/info/links/fda/regulations.aspx

www.meddramsso.com/MSSOWeb/index.htm

www.m-w.com/dictionary/quality%20control (Merriam-Webster's Online Dictionary)

www.m-w.com/dictionary/quality%20assurance (Merriam-Webster's Online Dictionary)

www.m-w.com/cgi-bin/dictionary?book=Dictionary&va=valid (Merriam-Webster's Online Dictionary)

www.m-w.com/cgi-bin/dictionary?book=Dictionary&va=verified (Merriam-Webster's Online Dictionary)

www.stylusinc.com/Common/Concerns/SoftwareDevtPhilosophy.php

Note: These urls were last accessed on 05MAR2008.

Index

Example Code — Examples from This Book at Your Fingertips

You can access the example programs for this book by linking to its companion Web site at **support.sas.com/companionsites**. Select the book title to display its companion Web site, and select **Example Code and Data** to display the SAS programs that are included in the book.

For an alphabetical listing of all books for which example code is available, see **support.sas.com/bookcode**. Select a title to display the book's example code.

If you are unable to access the code through the Web site, send e-mail to **saspress@sas.com**.

Comments or Questions?

If you have comments or questions about this book, you may contact the author through SAS as follows.

Mail: SAS Institute Inc.
SAS Press
Attn: <Author's name>
SAS Campus Drive
Cary, NC 27513

E-mail: saspress@sas.com

Fax: (919) 677-4444

Please include the title of the book in your correspondence.

See the last pages of this book for a complete list of books available through **SAS Press** or visit **support.sas.com/publishing**.

SAS Publishing News: Receive up-to-date information about all new SAS publications via e-mail by subscribing to the SAS Publishing News monthly eNewsletter. Visit **support.sas.com/subscribe**.

Lightning Source UK Ltd.
Milton Keynes UK
UKOW020737110313

207451UK00007B/189/P